ALICE HART-DAVIS
& BETH HINDHAUGH

100 WAYS FOR EVERY GIRL TO LOOK & FEEL FANTASTIC

WALKER BOOKS
AND SUBSIDIARIES

LONDON • BOSTON • SYDNEY • AUCKLAND

Contents

Clothes

Exercise

Wellbeing

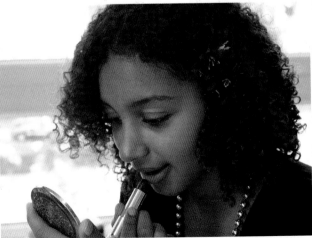

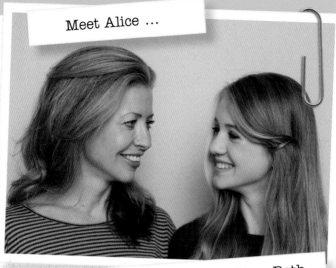

Meet Alice ...

... and her daughter, Beth.

Everyone wants to look great and feel fantastic. But how
do you go about it? And where do you start? This book
is here to give you a helping hand.

We've put together 100 tips and ideas to help you look
and feel your very best. You could try one of them, or you
could try all of them. Each one is a little step along the way
to being even more fantastic than you already are.

We really hope you enjoy this book – these ideas work
for us, and we hope they'll work for you, too.

With love,

Alice & Beth x

Face Care

How easy is it to have great skin? As easy as 1, 2, 3. Just keep it clean, keep it moisturized, and protect it from the sun. But what about spots? Read on to find out how to deal with them...

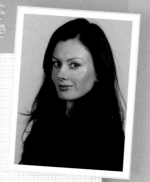

WHAT THE EXPERT SAYS

Dr Sam Bunting is a leading dermatologist, or skin specialist. She treats many young people (and sometimes their mums) for acne. Here are her top tips:

☑ **Cleanse gently.** Cleansers should get rid of make-up and excess oil – and that's it. Problems like dry skin or spots will be best treated with products you leave on your skin.

☑ **Stick with your spot treatment.** Red pimples and whiteheads will only benefit from two things: salicylic acid and benzoyl peroxide, the most effective anti-inflammatories around. Spot treatments take time to work so don't lose hope.

☑ **Protect yourself from the sun.** Wear sun protection, don't be tempted to use sunbeds and avoid strong sunlight between 11 a.m. and 3 p.m. Almost all the changes associated with looking older are due to sun exposure.

☑ **Know your skin type.** This will help you pick the right products (see tip, right).

☑ **See your good points.** Too often we focus on negative things and this can damage our self-esteem. It's important to be comfortable in your own skin.

1 get into a skincare routine

A regular routine using products that suit your skin type will help your skin stay smooth, clear and free from blemishes – no matter what life throws at it.

What your skin has to cope with

When you're inside, central heating or air conditioning can dry your skin out. When you're outside, sunshine bombards it with ultraviolet rays. Airborne pollution makes your skin dirty, and dirt can clog pores. If you're doing sport, you're going to sweat. At the same time, your skin produces sebum, its natural oil, and whenever you touch your face, bacteria from your fingers are added to the ones that naturally live on your skin. Get rid of all that gunk by cleansing and exfoliating, and give your skin a touch of moisture – your skin will thank you for it.

2 cleanse

Cleaning off all the oil, dirt, bacteria and make-up that builds up on your skin by the end of the day is the best thing you can do for your face. It will help keep your skin looking its natural best.

How to cleanse

♥ The kindest way to cleanse your face is with a cream or lotion. Massage it on with your fingers, then wipe it off with a flannel or muslin cloth rinsed out in warm water.

♥ Creamy cleansers are good for all skin types. They remove excess oil (so they're good for oily skin) without drying skin out (so they're good for dry skin, too).

♥ You don't have to wash your face until it's squeaky clean. That strips away all the skin's natural oils and makes your skin think it needs to produce more oil to restore the balance.

♥ Try not to scrub your face. It won't make it any cleaner but it could damage your skin and make it sore.

tip Dr Sam Bunting says: to work out your skin type, press some single-ply tissue on to your face an hour after cleansing, to see where the oily bits are. If there's oil on your forehead, nose and chin, you have combination skin. If there's no oil on the tissue, your skin is normal – but if your skin feels tight, it's dry. If there's oil all over, you have oily skin.

3 exfoliate

Your skin is constantly producing new cells which work their way to the top, die, and are shed. You never notice them go, unless they stick together and come off in flakes. Exfoliating clears away these old, dead cells, to keep your skin smooth and fresh-looking.

How to exfoliate

❤ Using a flannel or muslin cloth is a gentle way of exfoliating.

❤ You could also use an exfoliating face scrub. There are some that are designed to be used every day, but even if you only use a scrub once or twice a week, be kind to your skin and do it gently.

❤ If your skin is greasy, exfoliating will help keep your pores clear, so they're not blocked by excess oil.

❤ If your skin is dry, exfoliating makes the surface smoother, so that moisturizer sinks in more easily and is more effective.

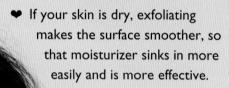

4 moisturize

Once your skin is clean, smooth and dry, it may feel a bit tight. If it does, you could do with a moisturizer.

How to moisturize

♥ Most skin types, except really oily ones, benefit from using moisturizer to help keep the skin supple and hydrated.

♥ If you have an oily T-zone (the area across your forehead and down the middle of your face), keep the moisturizer for the drier areas like your cheeks.

♥ Whatever your skin type, remember that oil and water are two different things. Your skin may be producing oil but that doesn't mean it doesn't need moisture.

♥ If your skin is dry, use a moisturizing cream.

♥ If your skin is normal, try a moisturizing lotion – this will be less heavy than a cream.

♥ If your skin is combination or oily, try an oil-free hydrating gel.

5 wear sunscreen

If you only put one thing on your face during the day, make it sunscreen. There are moisturizing sunscreens, oil-free sunscreens and tinted sunscreens, so there are plenty to choose from.

Why sunscreen is important

♦ Ultraviolet light – i.e. everyday daylight, not just sunlight – damages your skin. Over the past twenty years, many scientific studies have shown the ageing effects of daylight on the skin.

♦ These effects are small but they stack up over time and cause the vast majority of lines, wrinkles, pigment marks and age spots that bother older people. If your skin never saw the sun, it would stay surprisingly clear, smooth and line-free, apart from the wrinkles you get thanks to your genes and skin type – oily skin (and well-moisturized skin) wrinkles much less quickly than dry skin. Lines and wrinkles aren't a worry for you at the moment, but it's something to bear in mind for the future.

♦ Continued exposure to the sun increases your chances of developing skin cancer, and wearing sunscreen minimizes this risk.

Did you know?

♦ One bad sunburn doubles your risk of developing melanoma, an aggressive form of skin cancer.

♦ Melanoma is the second most common cancer in children and young adults.

♦ It's quite possible to get a sunburn if it's cloudy (the UVB rays, which tan and burn skin, pass through clouds).

These are facts and you should know them. You don't need to hide from the sun, but be careful. It's easy to protect your skin, and in the long term you'll be glad you did.

6 take action on spots

Most teenagers get spots, but that doesn't mean you have to put up with them. To a doctor, spots are a normal problem and there are a variety of solutions. So don't suffer: get help.

What causes spots?

Spots are mostly caused by the hormonal surges that hit you during puberty. They're not caused by eating the wrong foods or wearing make-up (though if your make-up is clogging your pores, it won't help).

How to beat spots

1. Get into the habit of cleansing your face properly, morning and night (see page 7). Start with gentle, non-medicated products that won't strip or irritate your skin. A regular routine of cleansing your skin and moisturizing any dry patches might be enough to keep your skin clear.

2. If this doesn't help, try using stronger, medicated anti-spot products that you can buy at the chemist. These contain either benzoyl peroxide, which dries out spots, or salicylic acid, which loosens the bonds that hold skin cells together, to prevent clumps of dead cells blocking your pores. Whatever you choose, use it consistently for six weeks.

3. If your spots persist, see your doctor – he or she can prescribe a stronger treatment for spots or refer you to a dermatologist.

Miracle cures for spots?

❤ **Blue light treatment**

This can help by killing the acne-causing bacteria on the skin, which will reduce the number of spots and help keep the skin clear. It doesn't treat the underlying hormonal causes of acne, but it makes spotty skin more manageable.

❤ **Roaccutane**

This is a very strong, prescription-only drug which a doctor or dermatologist may prescribe. It works by shrinking the oil-producing glands in the skin, which usually brings about a dramatic improvement in acne. On the down side, it makes the rest of your skin and your lips extremely dry, too. It shouldn't be given to anyone with a history of depression; some studies suggest it makes negative feelings much worse, although other studies suggest the opposite. Usually only one course of medication is needed.

tip Dr Sam Bunting says: to treat a spot, use a concealer in the morning which contains salicylic acid and is non-comedogenic (meaning it won't block pores). Then at night, clean the skin and apply a benzoyl peroxide-based spot cream (2.5% is strong enough). Then leave it alone and do not squeeze!

How Beth got the better of her spots

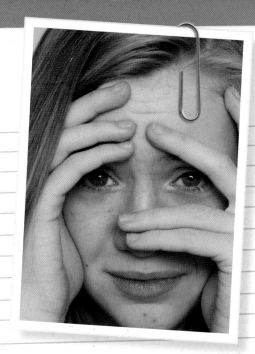

Q What's your main concern about your skin?

A I always seem to have spots, no matter what I use on my skin.

Q What sort of things have you tried?

A I've tried natural washes and anti-spot lotions which didn't do much, and I've tried stronger, medicated washes which left my skin sore and scaly … but still spotty.

Q So what did the trick? You don't look very spotty now…

A When everything I'd tried hadn't worked, I got an appointment with a dermatologist.

Q What did the dermatologist say?

A I wasn't particularly spotty when I went to see her, but she was very straightforward – she just said, "Why should you have to have ANY spots?" It was a relief to hear that. I thought you had to have tons of acne to see a dermatologist. I took the antibiotics she prescribed for three months and I also used special prescription creams. They've really made a difference, and my skin has improved a lot.

7 say no to cigarettes

Smoking will do a great deal of harm to your health and your skin – not to mention staining your teeth yellow and giving you bad breath.

Why smoking is bad for your skin

♦ Smoking ages your skin faster than anything except sun damage.

♦ One puff of cigarette smoke produces a trillion "free radical" particles in your lungs. These make skin old before its time.

♦ Nicotine is a stimulant and makes the blood vessels in your skin constrict: each cigarette stops the blood flowing through the tiny capillaries in your skin for twenty minutes. This deprives your skin of oxygen and so over time, smoking makes your skin look a bit yellow.

♦ Smokers' skin looks older faster. Studies have shown smoking ages the skin all over the body, not just on the face.

♦ Smoking strips skin of vitamin C, which is important for keeping the skin firm.

♦ Smoking dries your skin out.

♦ If you look at the skin of a smoker in her twenties under a microscope, you can see where early wrinkles will have started forming, even though none are visible to the naked eye.

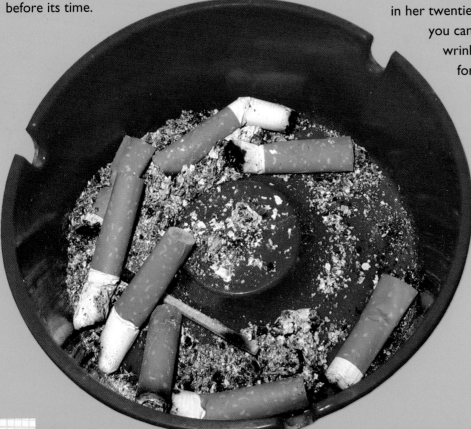

Make-up

Make-up doesn't have to be perfect —
it's meant to be fun. Experiment with
colour and texture, and try out different
looks. That way you can work out what
suits you best.

WHAT THE EXPERT SAYS

Louise Constad is a celebrity make-up artist. She created all of the make-up looks in this book. Here are her top tips:

☑ **Look at make-up as something to play with.** Go through magazines and tear out looks you like, for inspiration. Have a go at copying them and see if they suit you.

☑ **Use a brush for applying foundation.** Yes, you can get away with using your fingers or a sponge, but a brush will give you a smoother finish. Using a brush makes it easy to mix in a bit of moisturizer to give a more see-through finish, which is all that young skin needs.

☑ **Try lots of different make-up.** That way, you will work out what things you like, and what looks good on you.

☑ **Try red blusher.** It might sound odd but it suits every type of complexion. We all have red blood flowing through the capillaries near to the surface of our skin, so using a red blusher picks up on that natural, underlying colouring.

☑ **If you don't like any of it, don't worry.** There's no law that says just because you have two eyes, you have to wear eyeshadow...

8 only use foundation where you really need it

Creating a smooth, even complexion is always seen as the first step when putting on make-up. And so it should be – but be careful how you go about it.

Less is more

You might think you'll get the best results – and a flawlessly even face – if you use heaps of foundation to cover up every scrap of your skin, but doing that can leave your face looking blanked out and mask-like. Less is more when it comes to foundation, and this is especially true when you're young.

Conceal and go

Some make-up artists don't use foundation at all – they just use concealer, patting it on the areas they want to cover, such as blemishes, redness around the nose and chin, or shadows under the eyes. They'll dab on a little and blend it in, and then see what the effect is before they apply any more. If you try this, you'll see that you end up with a more natural-looking face, with minimal cover and more of your own skin on show.

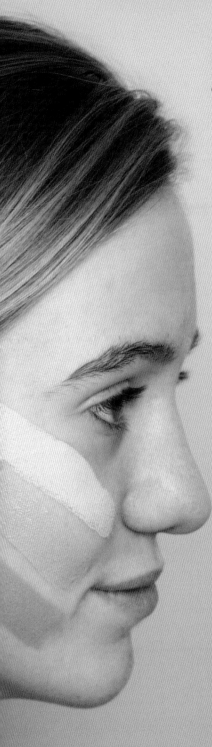

9 choose the right foundation

First you'll need to identify whether your skin tone has pinkish (cool) or yellowish (warm) undertones.

The colour test

The easiest way to work out whether you have warm or cool undertones is to put something gold, then something silver, against your face. One will suit you down to the ground; the other will make you look a bit drab. If the gold suits you better then you have "warm" skin; if the silver is better then you're "cool". Foundations which are more pink than yellow suit cool skin. Foundations which are more yellow than pink suit warm skin. Lots of people dab foundation on the inside of their wrist to see if it's the right colour. That's OK, but really you need to pop a bit on your face. This is where the cool-warm division really shows up. If you're "cool" and a foundation is "warm", it will look too yellow for your skin. When you find the right colour, it will seem to just vanish into your skin.

Types of foundation

	What it's like	Good for	Look for	Be careful
Liquid	Runny, so it comes in a bottle. Some give a thick, heavy, paste-like coverage, others are lighter and give a more sheer finish.	Giving a dewy finish to dry skin.	Reflective particles or "optical brighteners" which boost skin radiance.	If you have oily skin, it may need blotting with powder or special face-blotting papers.
Cream to powder	Comes as a solid, creamy block in a compact. Apply it with the sponge provided.	Carrying around with you (less likely to spill than a bottle). If you have a small brush, you can use it as concealer.	A light texture which is easy to spread.	If you have dry skin, it may have a drying effect or look patchy.
Mineral powder	A powder that you buff on with a brush, using firm, circular movements rather than up and down brush strokes.	Oily skin – the powder helps absorb the excess oil.	Built-in sunscreen. That means you're getting protection from harmful UV rays as well as skin-perfecting cover.	Make sure you buff it on as directed. If you just brush it lightly over your face, it won't give proper coverage.

10 learn how to use concealer

Concealer is a flesh-coloured paste (a bit like thicker foundation) designed to cover up flaws and blemishes.

Pick a colour as close to your skin tone as possible. Even better, find a concealer that offers you two colours in a single compact – then you can mix them until you have the right shade. Like foundation, concealer is either yellow-based or pink-based.

Cover your spots

Unless you have a special, medicated spot-concealer, apply a spot treatment gel to the spot before you start on the concealer, and let it dry. Using your finger or a small, flat-ended brush, pat concealer onto the spot to hide any redness, then blend the concealer into the surrounding skin. When you do the blending, add a tiny drop of moisturizer to the concealer to stop it going dry and looking cakey.

Disguise dark circles

Concealer is great for disguising dark circles under your eyes. The skin in this area is very thin and can get quite dry, so moisturize it before you start. You can pat the concealer on with a finger but you will get a smoother result if you use a small brush to apply it. Don't use too much – you don't want to look as if you've got white stripes under your eyes when you step back from the mirror.

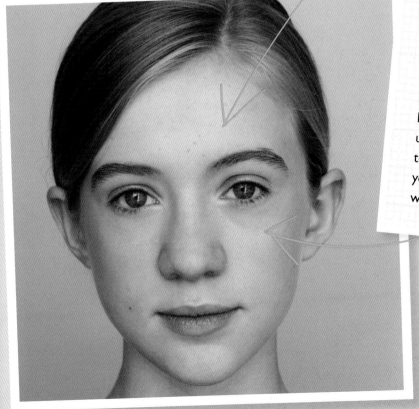

tip Use pink-based concealer to hide blueish dark smudges below your eyes. Then, if the colour looks all wrong, pat a little yellow-toned concealer over the top.

11 try out tinted moisturizer

Halfway between a foundation and a moisturizer, this does two jobs in one. You need to find one that's the right colour. It can be tempting to pick a product in the shade you'd like your skin to be, rather than the shade it actually is, but that way you may end up with a face that's a different colour from your neck and hands.

tip Find a tinted moisturizer with sun protection built in and you'll get protection from harmful UV rays, too. Look for "SPF" (short for "Sun Protection Factor" followed by a number (usually 15) on the tube.

12 get to grips with blusher

Blusher is brilliant for making your face look pretty and healthy, but it can be tricky to use. If you use too little, it will hardly show and you'll wonder why you bothered, but if you use too much, you can end up looking like a

doll with painted-on cheeks. All you need to do is practise, to see what looks right for you. It will be well worth the effort.

How to apply cream blusher

1. Find as bright a light as you can. If you apply blusher in a dim light, you'll use more blusher to see an effect. When you emerge into the daylight you'll find you've made your cheeks far too colourful.

2. Smile, then dab a spot of colour onto the "apples" of your cheeks (these are the bits that bunch up when you smile).

3. Using your finger, blend this colour into an oval shape, up along your cheekbone and towards the side of your face.

How to apply powder blusher

Once you've got used to how you look wearing blusher, experiment with powder blusher. These usually come with a tiny brush which is pretty useless; what you need is a big, soft blusher brush.

1. Sweep up a bit of colour onto the brush and tap the brush to shake off any excess.

2. Smile, and land the colour on the apples of your cheeks, sweeping it back towards your temples.

3. Blend it in like mad before you add any more colour and keep checking in the mirror that you have an even effect on both cheeks.

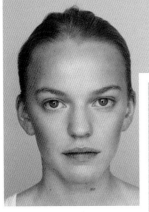

Statement look

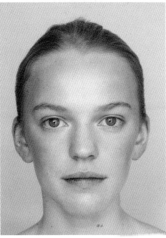

Natural look

13 look healthy with bronzer

Bronzer is a brownish powder that comes in a flat compact. It is best to put it on with as big a brush as you can find, and use it to give your face a hint of colour.

How to apply bronzer

For best results, you need to use it cleverly, rather than just spreading it all over your face like a self-tan.

1. Imagine you're tilting your face up to the sun, and think of the parts that would catch the sun the most – the bridge of your nose, your cheekbones and forehead, and your chin. These are the areas to start with.

2. Swipe the brush lightly across the bronzer, tap off any excess, then dust it onto your face. Use it lightly to start with until you can see the effect it's having. It's easy to brush it on and find that you've got a thick stripe of colour which is hard to blend in.

3. Finish off by dusting a tiny bit of bronzer into the edges of your face at your hairline, and around your chin.

tip Bronzer or blusher? Blusher is pink, red or orange, and just used on the cheeks. Bronzer is tan, bronze or brown, and can be used all over the face. If you use both at once, you may look overly made-up, so go for one or the other.

Blusher

Natural look

Statement look

19

Make-up

14 learn new looks with eyeliner

Using eyeliner is one of the easiest ways to emphasize your eyes. You could stick to plain, bold black, try a light or bright colour as a lively contrast to the colour of your eye, or choose a softer shade that echoes your eye colour and makes it stand out.

Different looks to try

1. Cleopatra: a line all around the eye with neat points at either end.

2. Up and over: a clean line with a downward sweep and no tail.

3. High fashion: a long, thin line which elongates the eye, echoed on the socket of the eye.

4. Colour flick: a classic flick, in colour.

5. Sixties flick: a neat line with a tidy flick.

6. Gold gleam: gold adds a bright accent.

7. Long tick: a thick outer edge and lengthened line make the eye look wider.

8. Fishtail flicks: lines along the upper and lower lids which don't meet at the corners.

9. The hook: a hook-shaped line helps define the inner corner of the eye.

10. Party party: electrifying statement flicks.

11. Silver sweep: silver on top and purple below.

12. Soft and sooty: liner inside and outside the lashes.

13. Thick flick: a heavyweight among flicks.

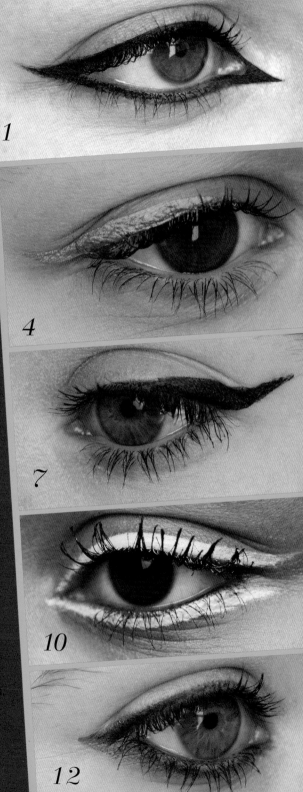

1

4

7

10

12

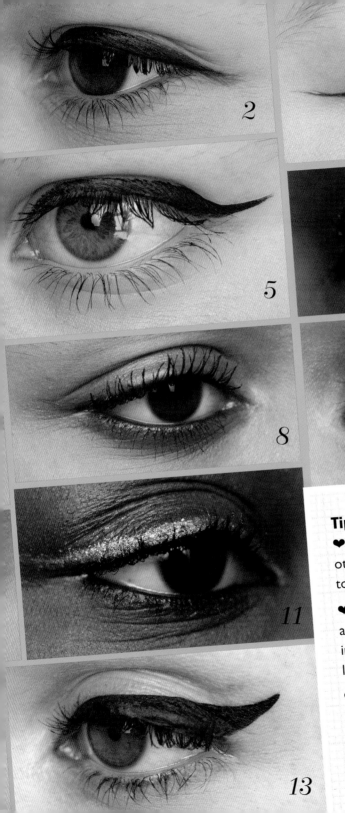

2

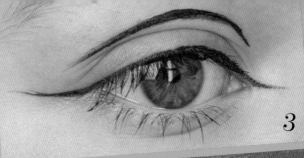

3

5

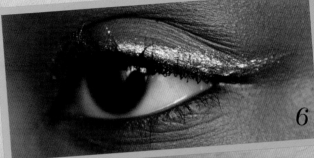

6

8

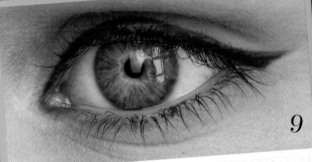

9

11

13

Tips for applying eyeliner

♥ Hold the eyelid taut with the fingers of your other hand, which gives you a steadier surface to draw on.

♥ Keep the liner as close to your eyelashes as possible. If you're using a pencil liner, work it in among the roots of your lashes, to make the lashline look thicker.

♥ Black eyeliner is hard on fair complexions. Try brown, green or bright colours; smudge them gently for a new take on smoky eyes.

♥ To "wake up" eyes, run a skin-coloured eyeliner along the inner rim of your lower lashes.

15 play with coloured eyeshadows

Neutral eyeshadows have their place, but colour says "time to party!" Purple and lilac set off blue eyes, green adds depth to hazel eyes, metallic shadows make dark eyes glow and contrasting eyeliner adds a punch of colour ... but there are no rules. See what suits your eyes and your mood.

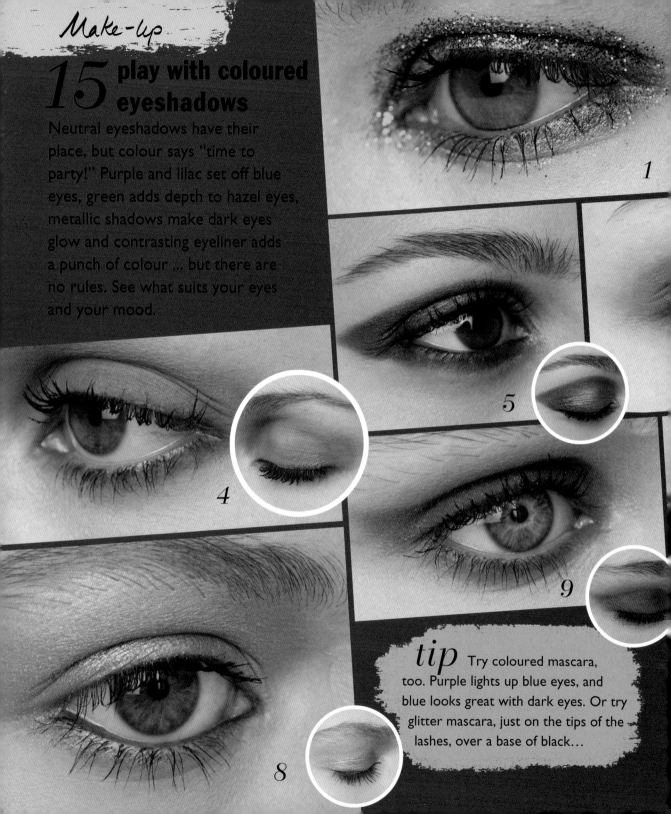

1

5

4

9

tip Try coloured mascara, too. Purple lights up blue eyes, and blue looks great with dark eyes. Or try glitter mascara, just on the tips of the lashes, over a base of black…

8

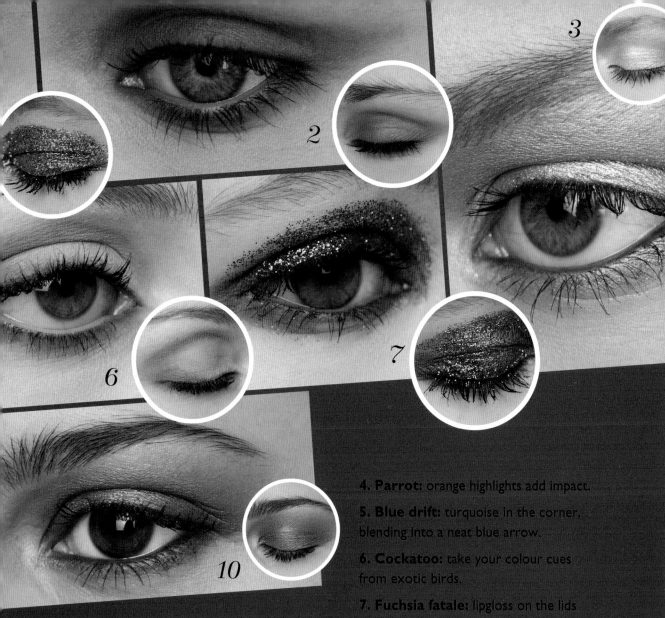

4. Parrot: orange highlights add impact.

5. Blue drift: turquoise in the corner, blending into a neat blue arrow.

6. Cockatoo: take your colour cues from exotic birds.

7. Fuchsia fatale: lipgloss on the lids helps the glitter to stick.

8. Solid gold: one-shade wonder, with contrasting liner.

9. Deep purple: blue liner works beautifully with rich mauve.

10. Modern metal: low-key metallic.

1. Glitter peacock: blue below the eye, and green above.

2. Purple arrow: perfect for blue-eyed girls.

3. Silver leaf: extra-intense shadow on the lid, blended into the brows.

23

16 curl your eyelashes

Curling your eyelashes is one of those simple things that really makes a difference – it instantly makes your eyes look prettier and more open. You need to curl your lashes before you put on mascara, not after. The mascara should then dry into the curl that you've created and help it to set.

How to curl your eyelashes

You will need an eyelash curler – a complicated little gadget with scissor-like handles that operate a metal clamp with rubberized pads.

1. Looking down, manoeuvre the eyelash curler so that its jaws are either side of your upper eyelashes.

2. Cautiously squeeze the curler shut. Ideally, you want it to grip all along your upper lashes, as close to the roots as possible. Do it slowly so you don't catch your eyelid in the pads – that really hurts.

3. Squeeze the curlers tightly for ten seconds, then carefully release. Your eyelashes should be noticeably curled.

tip To enhance the curling effect, heat the curlers for a few seconds with a hairdryer before you use them. (Be careful – don't heat them too much!)

17 experiment with false eyelashes

False lashes are fiddly but when you want to make a statement they can be very effective. There are all sorts of different kinds. The lashes shown here are fabulously over the top. Choose more natural-looking falsies for a gentler kind of eyelash enhancement.

Buy more than one pair at first, just in case one of them goes wrong. If you can, buy a tube of special eyelash glue, too. There will be a tiny tube supplied with the lashes, but it's not always the best-quality stuff.

How to put on false eyelashes

False lashes should go on after you've done your eyeshadow, so do that first, and then apply the lashes. Take your time.

1. Remove one eyelash and hold it up along your lashes. It will probably be too long, so measure how much you want to reduce it by, then cut a bit off the end that will go nearest your nose. Measure this against the other lash and trim that one down, too.

2. Spread a thin line of glue along the edge of the lash strip. If there's no brush supplied, use a toothpick or a matchstick. You can use your finger, but wipe it clean before you apply the lash, otherwise you may end up with the lash glued to your finger rather than your eyelid.

3. Let the glue dry for five seconds so that it becomes tacky, then carefully position the lash along your lashline, as close to the roots of your natural lashes as you can. Press it down in the middle then work towards the inner corner of your eye. Then, from the centre, work outwards to the outer corner. When it's all in place, keep your fingers over the outer and inner ends of the lash for another thirty seconds, to stick it extra-firmly (the ends are always the first bits to work themselves loose). If it doesn't end up sticking exactly along the lash-line, use liquid eyeliner to paint over the join and hide it.

4. To mesh the false lashes in with your own, add a coat of mascara – a normal, non-volumizing mascara works best for this. If the lashes look a bit claggy, comb them through with an old (washed and dried) mascara wand.

5. When the party's over, don't rip the lashes off and throw them away – you can re-use them. Peel them off carefully and put them away in the little tray that they came in.

tip Some brands that sell false eyelashes, particularly the ones in department stores, will also fix them on for you. It's always worth asking.

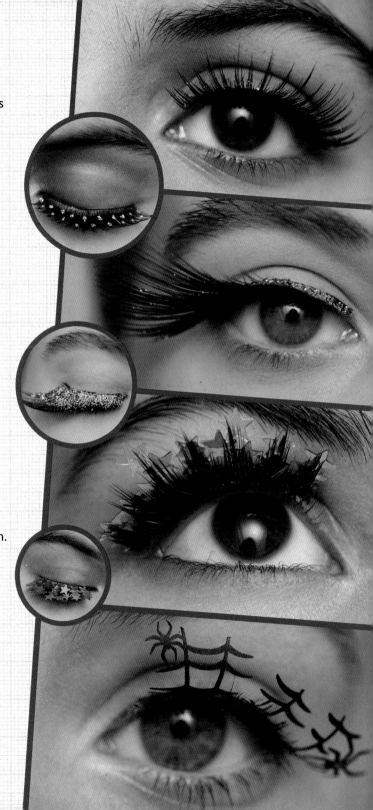

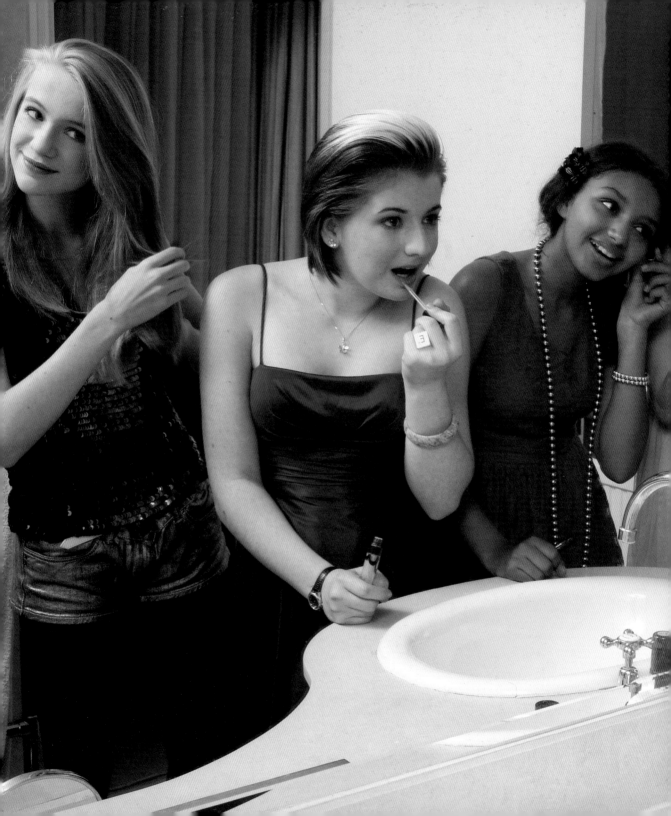

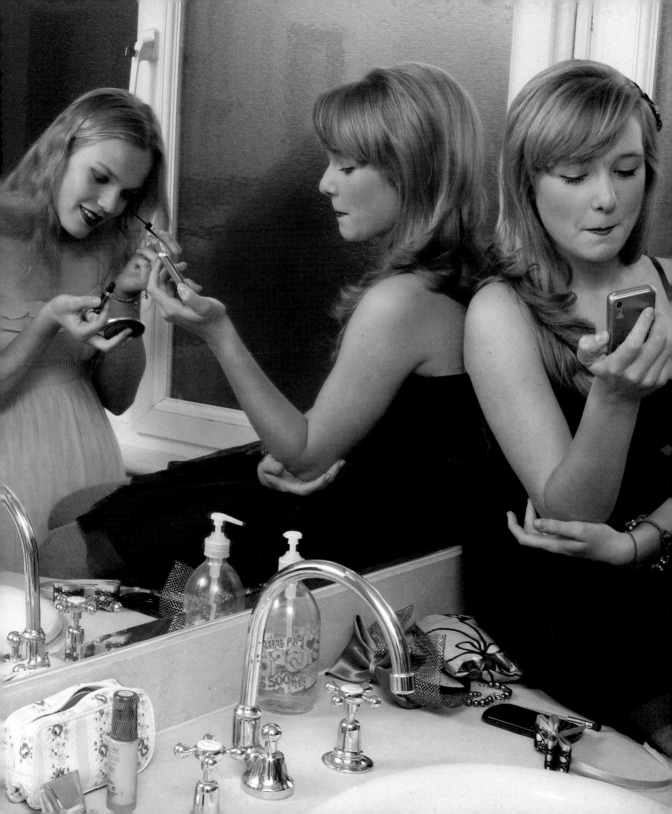

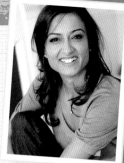

WHAT THE EXPERT SAYS

Shavata Singh is an A-list eyebrow guru. Here are her top tips:

☑ **Use a brow-shape stencil.** You can buy these as kits and they can help you with the basic shape.

☑ **Use good-quality tweezers.** They help you to get a better grip on each hair.

☑ **Tweeze your eyebrows after a hot bath or shower.** It's best to pluck them in natural daylight, too.

☑ **Just take a few hairs at a time from each side.** This is much easier than doing one whole brow then trying to copy it on the other side.

☑ **Think of your eyebrows as sisters, not twins.** No one has identical eyebrows, so don't try to force yours to be exactly the same as each other.

☑ **Don't pluck too many hairs from the inner edges of your eyebrows.** The inside end of your eyebrow should start above the inner corner of your eye.

☑ **Only pluck hairs from underneath your brows.** Never pluck from above.

☑ **Stick to basic shaping and tidying.** If you pluck them too much, those hairs may never grow back.

18 shape your eyebrows

Making your eyebrows look neat and defined can improve your look massively. The easiest way to start is by getting your eyebrows shaped professionally (this would be a great present – it's not expensive). Then you can stick to this shape by tweezing away any stragglers as they grow back.

Using brow stencils

1. Find a stencil in a shape you like – but make sure it's reasonably similar to your own eyebrow shape (if you have high, arched brows, you're never going to get them to look flat and bushy).

2. Holding the stencil over each of your eyebrows in turn, mark in the outline of the brow shape you're after with an eyebrow pencil or eyeliner pencil. It's easier if you get a friend to help.

3. Work out where you need to make changes and do it slowly, taking only a few hairs from each side alternately.

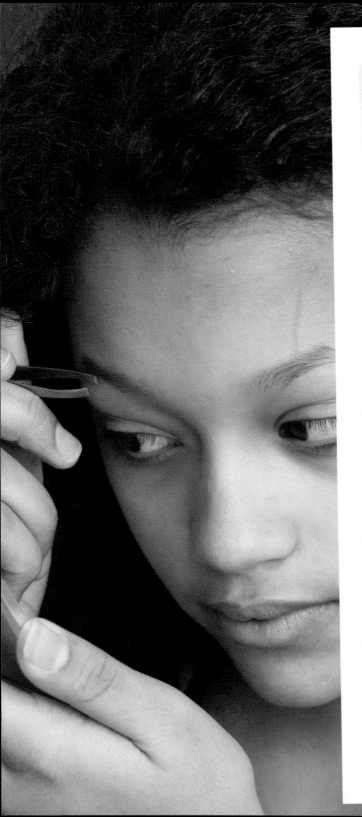

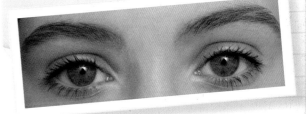

Beth gets her eyebrows shaped

Q How did you feel about having your eyebrows shaped?

A I was a bit nervous – I'd never plucked my eyebrows before, and I'd been told it really hurts.

Q So what was it like?

A It was painful, even though Louise (the make-up artist who plucked them for me) was very quick with the tweezers. She said one eyebrow always hurts more than the other.

Q Are you pleased with the result?

A Yes. My brows don't look drastically different but I can see they look neater.

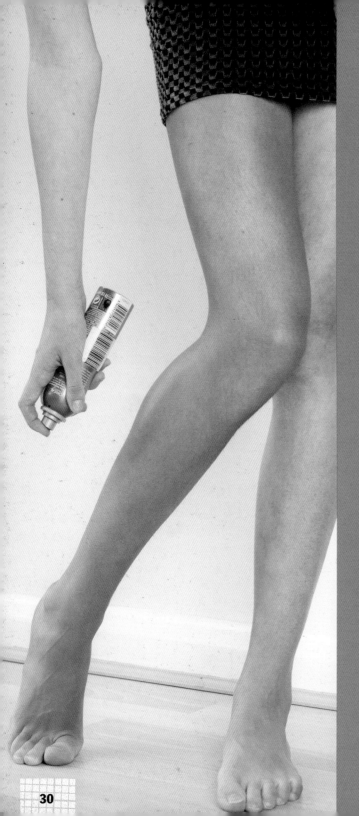

19 become a self-tan fan

No matter how many times beauty magazines tell us that pale is beautiful, the urge to tan is as strong as ever – but it's much better for the health of your skin to fake a tan than to roast your skin in the sun.

Build it up

It's easiest to build up the colour by using a gradual-tan formula. These look like everyday, cream-coloured lotions, and rub in easily. They contain a low level of the same tanning ingredient as stronger tanning products.

Which formula to use

Should you use a cream? A mousse? A gel? Whichever you like. These are all easy to use formulas, especially if the product is tinted so that you can see where you've applied it. The really runny liquid tints are harder to handle.

You may need to try a few different products until you find one that produces a realistic colour on your skin.

How to use self-tan

Whichever product you use, the principles are the same.

1. Exfoliate all over first. This will get rid of dry, scuffy bits of dead skin. That means the product will sink in more evenly wherever you apply it, so you should end up with a smoother result.

2. Before you start with the product, put some moisturizing lotion on your elbows, wrists, knees, feet, ankles and the backs of your hands. The skin is thinner and drier on these bits, and moisturizing first will stop the self-tan from sinking in more quickly and ending up darker on these areas.

3. Apply the product quickly and evenly, and give yourself time to dry off before you get dressed. While you're drying off, wash your hands really thoroughly – you don't want tan stains on your palms. But bear in mind that if you wash all the self-tan off the backs of your hands, you may end up with a tan that stops at your wrists. So, either don't wash the backs of your hands, or apply a smidgen more tan here after you've washed them.

4. Fake tan takes a while to work, and gets browner on your skin – don't apply too much, thinking that it's not working.

Skin finishing

There's a new art to making bare limbs look fantastic. Make-up artists call it "skin finishing". It's less about being toasty-brown and more about getting limbs glowing. For a pale gold glow, massage in a dry body oil or gel-oil – some have gold or glitter for added sparkle. To give your legs and arms a gleam of bronze, sweep on some bronzing gel or brush-on bronzing powder. The best thing is you can wash it off afterwards.

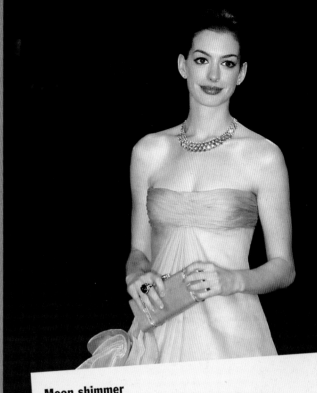

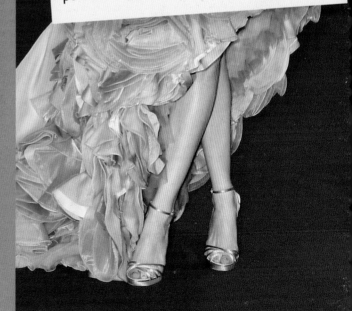

Moon shimmer
If you've got beautifully pale skin like Anne Hathaway, embrace it. Ditch the self-tan and use a skin illuminator gel or shimmering dusting powder to give yourself an ethereal sheen.

20 use make-up brushes

Which ones do you really need? And what do you need them for? That depends on what sort of make-up you wear.

1. A big blusher/ powder brush

Use it lightly. Dip it in powder, or dash it across your blusher, then tap it to make sure that there isn't too much powder on it. For blusher blend it up over your cheekbones; for powder buff it round in light circles, so that the powder settles onto your face.

2. A small eyeshadow brush

Just brush up some eyeshadow from the palette, and go play.

3. An eyeliner/eyebrow brush

Eyeliner: press the angled end flat into your eyeliner (or eyeshadow), then press this closely above your upper lashes, or below your lower lashes. Start at the inner corner of your eye, and work outwards. Use the brush to blend the line into the lash roots.

Eyebrows: to emphasize eyebrows, dust a little eyeshadow, just a bit darker than your natural eyebrow colour, onto the brush. Then brush this through your eyebrows, following the direction the hairs grow in.

4. A foundation brush

Put some liquid foundation on the back of your hand. Work the brush into this and then use the brush to paint the foundation lightly onto your skin, spreading it out as thinly as you can. Start with the areas that most need a bit of coverage and use as little foundation as you can get away with.

5. A lip brush

Dip the brush into your lipstick until it has a decent amount of colour on it, then, starting with your top lip, draw in the outline of your lips. Use what's left on the brush to sketch in some colour on the body of your lips, then fill this bit in with more lipstick.

6. A concealer brush

Put a little concealer on the back of your hand. Dip the tip of your brush into the concealer and dab it lightly where it's needed.

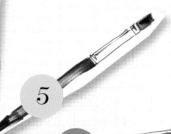
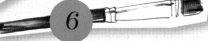

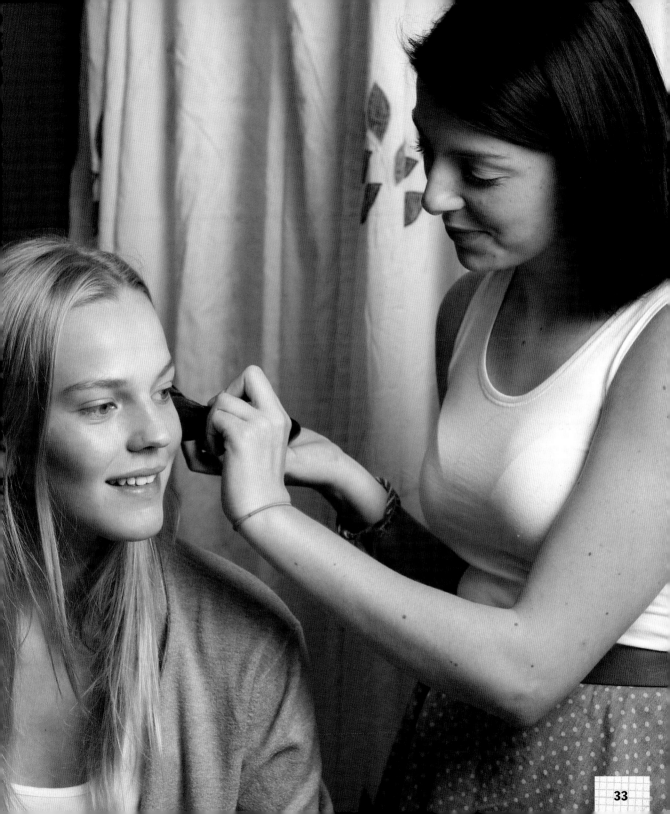

21 use less lip balm

Seriously, it can become addictive – the more you use it, the more you need to use it. Lip balm forms a layer that stops moisture escaping through the thin skin on the lips. This will keep your lips from drying out, but it will also slow down the natural process by which the drying-out of lips prompts your skin to push up new, fresh skin cells from underneath. So cut down on lip balm. After all, boys get by without it most of the time…

22 soften your lips

Get rid of dead, flaky skin on your lips with this time-honoured method.

How to exfoliate your lips

First smother your lips in balm to soften the dead skin. Then use an old toothbrush to rub off the balm and the dead skin (it's gentler on your lips if you run the toothbrush under hot water first, to soften the bristles).

Even better, use a lip-exfoliating scrub or sugar to do the job – this is kinder to the delicate skin on your lips. Again, apply lip balm, then rub a pinch of sugar over your lips (if your lip balm is a twist-up one, you can just dunk it in sugar, then rub it on).

23 rock those lips

Try these lip looks to see what works for you.

1. **Fluoro pink:** looks great if you've got blue eyes.

2. **Blackout:** go as dark as you dare to be right on trend.

3. **Orange brights:** punchy and colourful, a hot look any time of year.

4. **Innocent pink:** a sweet and natural look.

5. **Two-tone:** chocolate lip-pencil teamed with baby-beige lipstick. For even more impact, try an orange outline filled in with bright pink.

6. **Classic red:** always a knockout. Keep it matte to keep it fashionable.

7. **Wildcat:** a quick-to-apply lip transfer gives the most startling results of all.

8. **Two-tone two:** electric blue and purple is an attention grabber.

tip If you're blessed with naturally huge lips and want to play them down, choose a dark lipstick, or a matt lip colour, or both. Dark, matt lipsticks don't reflect light, so they will make your lips seem smaller than they are.

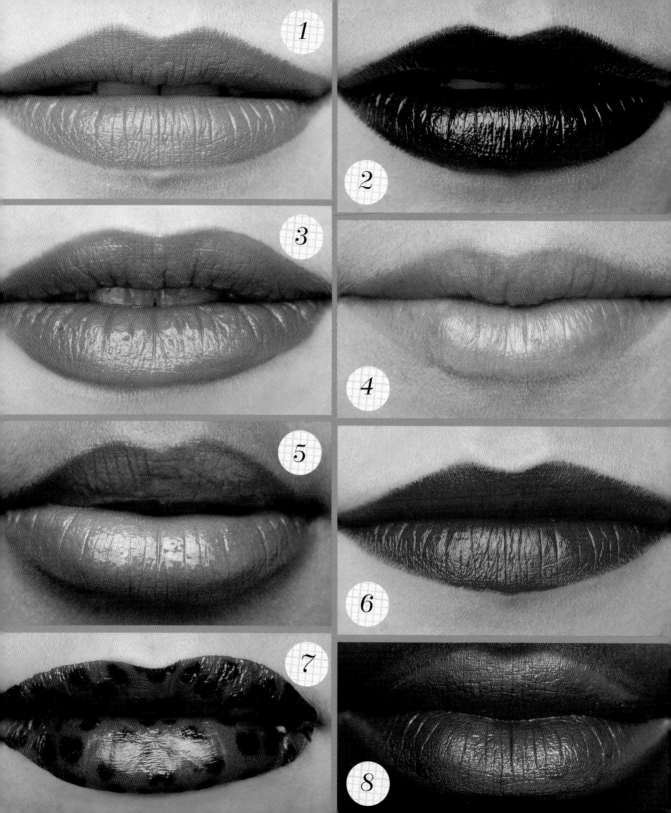

24 find a signature look

Examine pictures of celebrities and you'll see that most have a particular make-up look that they turn to time and time again, because it works so well. Here are their secrets.

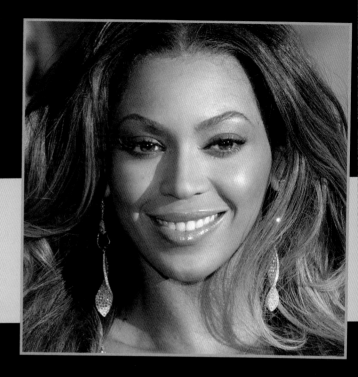

Colourful eyes – Beyoncé

Beyoncé never lets her eyes fade into the background. For a party, try wearing bright colours around your eyes – pinks, blues, or whatever works with what you're wearing.

Glamorous, smoky eyes – Adele

Adele is rarely seen without smoky eyes and a flick of eyeliner – a sultry look which isn't too hard to copy. The easiest way to create a smoky eye is to use just one colour of eyeshadow. Apply it generously to the eyelid, and then use a brush to blend the colour softly all the way up to the brow bone. Finish off with a flicky line of liquid eyeliner.

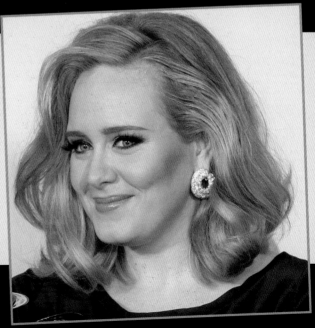

Strong eyebrows – Emma Watson

Even when she's wearing almost no make-up, Emma's distinctive eyebrows frame her face and her large eyes beautifully. If you aren't blessed with such naturally great brows, you can give yours more oomph with an eyebrow pencil. Pick a shade slightly darker than your natural brow colour, and work along each brow in turn using short, feathery strokes.

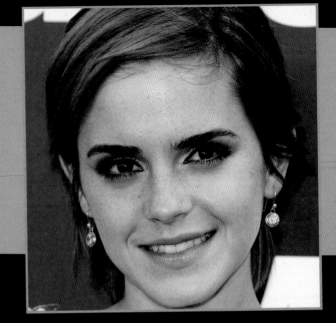

A fresh-faced glow – Selena Gomez

To get your skin looking gorgeously fresh without smothering it in make-up, mix a dab of moisturizer in with some foundation on the back of your hand and blend this over your face. The foundation will give your skin an even tone, and the moisturizer will keep it light and dewy. If you find your face is threatening to look more oily than dewy, press face-blotting paper (or, at a pinch, a tissue, pulled in half so it's extra-thin) gently over your face. That way you keep the glow without the shine.

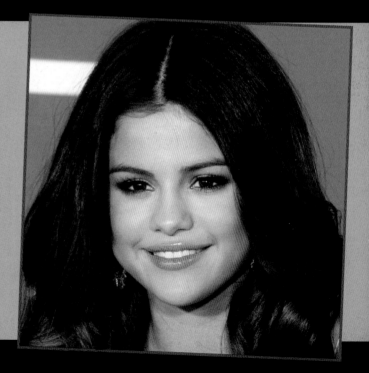

25 make your make-up do double duty

Make-up artists are great at making their products work hard for them – they use them all in a variety of ways. You can do the same.

Try using...

Mascara to colour your eyebrows. This is best done with a clean, separate mascara wand, as you need very little mascara to make an impact on your brows. Comb it through and tidy up any smudges with a cotton bud.

Use concealer instead of foundation. Just dab it on the areas that really need it.

Use lip balm on your eyelids. It will give you a super glossy finish. Use it on bare lids for a summery shine, or wipe it over eye shadow for a glam look.

Use eye shadow as eyeliner. You'll need a small, stiff brush with a rectangular end. Dip the brush in water, then dab it on the shadow. Use the wet shadow as liner, pressing it carefully along the lash line.

Use cheek colour on your lips. And vice versa. There are plenty of lip-and-cheek stains specially designed to be used on both.

If you're really travelling light...

… you could get away with one creamy, pinky-brown lipstick.

❤ Dot it on your cheeks and blend, as blusher.

❤ Spread a smidgen of it on your brow bones (the bones beneath your eyebrows) to make your eyes pop.

❤ Blend a tiny bit on the point of your chin, the tip of your nose and your hairline, where you would use a bronzer.

❤ Then gloss up your lips with it – and you're all set.

26 take your make-up off every night

It's really important for the health of your skin to take your make-up off at night. During the day your skin will have picked up dirt, sweat, bacteria and oil, and you need to get rid of that as well as your make-up.

1. Start by taking the worst of it off with a cleansing wipe.

2. Massage a cleanser over your skin.

3. Wipe the cleanser off with a flannel wrung out in hot water.

4. Finish with a dab of moisturizer. Then your skin can breathe again.

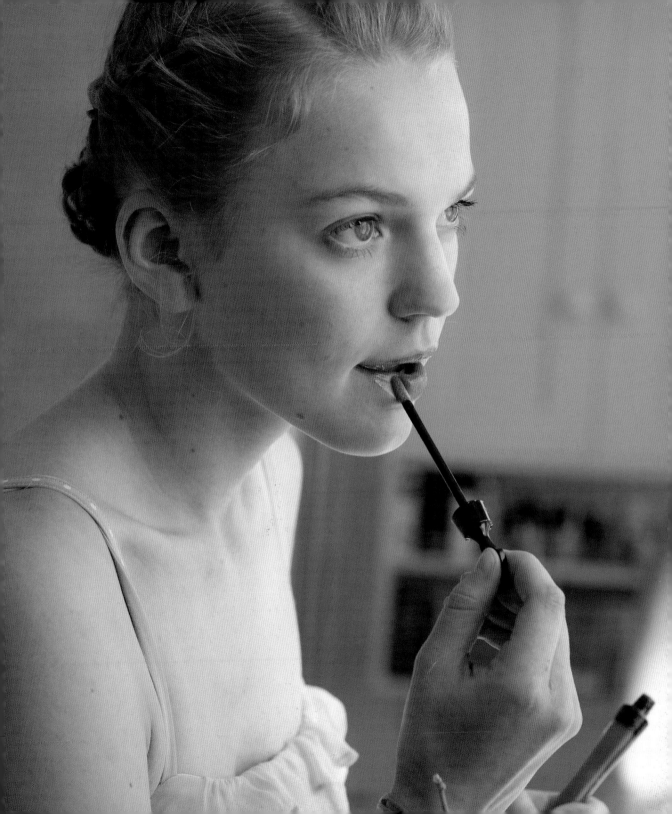

Beth's favourite
make-up look

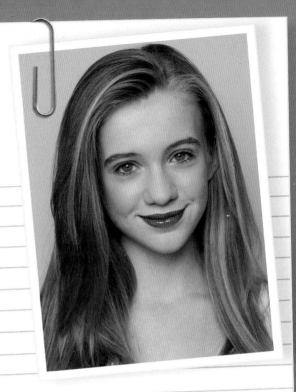

Q **What's your favourite make-up trick at the moment?**

A I love wearing bright lip colours. I first tried using a red lip stain – it feels more fun and less grown-up than lipstick.

Q **Did you wear it for parties?**

A No, I wore it at school. I felt like a bit of an idiot when I put it on in front of people because it comes in an applicator that looks like a red felt pen – it looked as if I was literally colouring in my lips. But once it was on, it stayed put and didn't smudge, and I really liked the way it looked.

Q **So what do you particularly like about this look?**

A Wearing a bright colour like this really does lift my mood. And if I'm having a bad hair day or my skin isn't great, putting the emphasis on my lips draws attention away from the rest of my face.

Q **So is bright red your signature look now?**

A I've found that bright pinks work well on me, too. But I don't have bright lips the whole time. It wouldn't be special if I did it every day.

Hair

Your hair should be your crowning glory.
How you wear it says a lot about how you
see yourself. Here's how to find a haircut
that suits you and style it brilliantly –
and avoid bad hair days for good.

Hair

27 get strong, healthy hair

We all want strong, thick, shiny, healthy-looking hair. Here's how to keep yours in the best condition.

Eat protein

Your hair is made of keratin, which is protein, and you need to eat plenty of protein to keep it strong — meat, fish, eggs, cheese, nuts and seeds are all good sources of protein.

Brush your hair

Brush it gently and don't drag a comb through it when it's wet. Start at the bottom when teasing out a mass of tangles, and work slowly.

Use conditioner

This smoothes down the hair cuticle and makes it less likely to snag when you brush it.

Use heat-protective sprays

Spritz them on before using hot styling appliances like straighteners or wands.

Protect your hair when swimming

Wet your hair before swimming in a chlorinated pool. Hair absorbs water, but if it's already full of tap water it won't absorb the chlorine that can damage and roughen it.

Get regular trims

If you get split ends, get them cut off. No treatment on earth will mend them. Think about what might be causing the split ends, too — it could be over styling, or rough brushing...

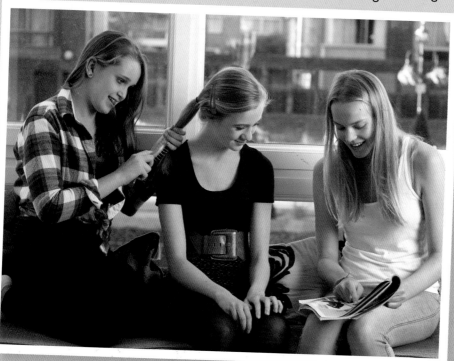

28 cut your hair

A haircut is one of the quickest ways to make a dramatic difference to the way you look, especially if you take a risk and have lots of it cut off.

Before you take the plunge

Talk through what you want to have done with your hairdresser. It's always easier if you bring in a picture of the look you're after. Your hairdresser should be able to give you an opinion on whether it will suit you or not. Make sure you are clear on all the details before they start. If you've said "with a fringe", what sort of fringe are you talking about (long and side-swept, chunky, wispy)?

How to find a good hairdresser

Ask around. Ask your friends, ask your mum, ask anyone whose hairstyle you like. If you can, have a brief chat with the stylist before jumping into their chair. If you aren't sure about them, or you don't like their personal style, trust your instincts and go elsewhere. It's your hair and your money, so you're entitled to be choosy.

If you have a bad haircut, it's best to shout a bit, cry a bit, and then get over it. Your hair will grow again.

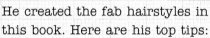

WHAT THE EXPERT SAYS

Mathew Alexander is a leading hairdresser with his own salon in London's West End. He created the fab hairstyles in this book. Here are his top tips:

☑ **Research the haircuts that you like.** If you like a particular celebrity's hairstyle, check that it looks good when they're out shopping as well as when it has been dressed for a special event. You don't want a cut that only looks good when it has been professionally styled.

☑ **Save up for a great cut.** Go for the best stylist you can afford – it will be worth it.

☑ **Become a hair model.** Ask the top salons in your area if they're looking for cutting models. You'll get your hair cut by a trainee who is being guided by an experienced stylist. Make sure you're clear about what you want and expect the haircut to take longer than a haircut done by an experienced stylist.

☑ **Ask your stylist for advice.** An experienced stylist will advise you about which styles will suit your face shape and your hair texture, and which won't.

29 try a dramatic change

Cutting your hair short is a bold move and can feel liberating – especially if you've got used to hiding behind long hair. Not only is this haircut much shorter but it has gone from dark blonde to dark brown.

tip Hair grows at around 15 cm a year, or 1.25 cm a month, so if you cut it pixie short, it will be a while before it has grown down to your shoulders again.

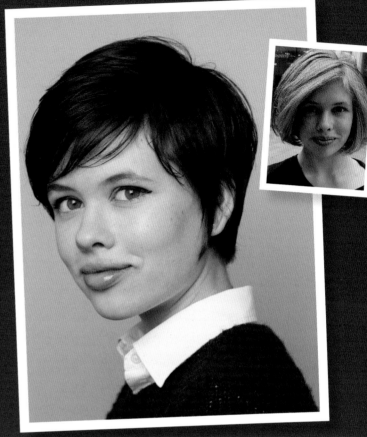

30 find the haircut that's right for you

A great haircut can make you feel on top of the world. Finding one that works for you depends on your face shape, your attitude, and how much time you want to spend styling it.

What's flattering?

"An oval face-shape can get away with any haircut," says Mathew Alexander, "so when hairdressers cut hair, they use layering and styling techniques to make the face look closer to an oval shape. A round face will need longer layers around the face and height in the hair to lengthen the face and a square face needs a style that will soften it, rather than a jaw-length bob or a squared-off fringe."

Fringe

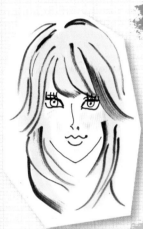

Pros: anyone can wear one. A good hairdresser can advise whether yours should be short, long, heavy or feathery.
Cons: a heavy fringe can make square faces look squarer and round faces wider.

Bob

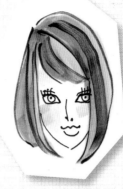

Pros: simple, chic, always fashionable. Can be long or short, worn with a fringe or without…
Cons: not very versatile. Needs regular cuts to keep it looking sharp.

Shag

Pros: adaptable. It's a rough-layered style with attitude that can be cut to suit any face shape.
Cons: it's rough and ready, so not great if you need to look conventionally smart.

Mid-length layers

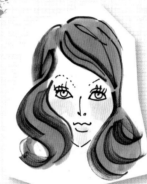

Pros: easy to wear and to adapt in various ways.
Cons: needs a bit of attention when blow-drying to make the most of it.

Pixie cut

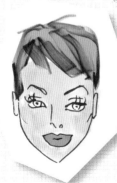

Pros: bound to turn heads. Can look cute, as long as you have the features to carry it off. Very easy to look after – it takes seconds to wash and dry.
Cons: very exposing (there's nothing to hide behind). Few ways to dress it up or make it different.

Long hair

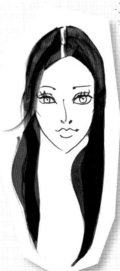

Pros: it's always impressive to have a lovely curtain of long hair. A safe option, particularly if most of your friends have hair like this. There's plenty you can do to dress it up.
Cons: not exactly a hairstyle as such. Can be a bit dull.

Hair
31 colour your hair

If you want to dye your hair, you can either pay for highlights, lowlights or a whole new head of colour at a hair salon, or buy a box of hair dye and do it yourself.

Having your hair dyed professionally will give you a more sophisticated, natural-looking and possibly less exciting result.

If you dye your hair at home – well, it's up to you. Go as wild as you like. But before you start, bear these bits of advice in mind.

Hair dye

There are two main types of dye: permanent and semi-permanent.

1. Permanent ... means permanent.

♥ The dye uses ammonia to fix colour deep in the cortex of the hair – the bit that gives hair its strength, flexibility and colour.

♥ It won't wash out and will give you the most dramatic colour change, but that means root regrowth will be really obvious.

♥ To create a statement without committing to a full colour change, try dyeing or bleaching a small section of hair. A chunk or streak near your face will be plain for all to see; a section near the ends of your hair will be easier to hide if you don't like the results.

2. Semi-permanent ... lasts for around six weeks.

♥ Uses the same chemicals as permanent dye, but at lower levels, so it doesn't last as long.

♥ Less drastic than permanent dye but will still give long-lasting colour.

Highlights

Taking strands of hair and dyeing them a few shades lighter than your natural colour, so it looks as if you've spent lots of time outside in the sun. Hard to do on yourself, because you can't see round to treat the back your head.

Lowlights

Taking strands of hair and dyeing them a few shades darker than your natural colour, to add variety and depth to your hair colour. If you don't want to dye your hair, try clipping in a few darker hair extensions to create instant lowlights. You could try lighter extensions to create highlights, too.

Blonding sprays

A mild form of hair bleach, which will lighten up the bits you spray it on.

Coloured hair sprays

The easiest way to liven up your hair colour temporarily. Try spraying the ends of your hair for a dip-dyed look.

Always do a patch test

Hair dye can cause severe allergic reactions, so before you use any kind of hair colour, do a patch test – try the dye on a small area of skin, 24 hours before you use it for real.

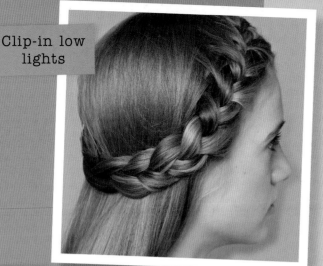

Clip-in low lights

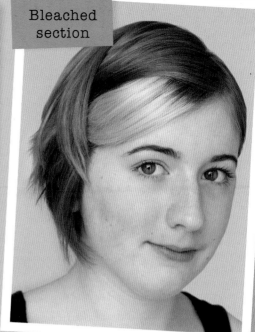

Bleached section

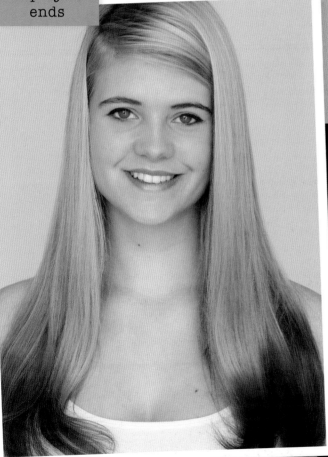

Dip-dyed ends

Things to bear in mind

Unless your hair is jet black, its natural colour will contain a variety of different shades, so dyeing it one solid colour will make it look a bit fake.

When you use a chemical colourant on your hair, you remove some of its natural protective coating. Once your hair is coloured, you'll need to condition it thoroughly and brush it more carefully, because it won't be as strong as it was before.

When your hair grows, the regrowth – your original hair colour – will show at the roots. You'll either need to keep dyeing it or put up with two-tone hair as it grows out.

Hair

32 style it!

If you put in the time to learn a few basic hair styling techniques, you'll be able to use them to create whichever of the latest looks takes your fancy. Here are three hairstyles to try.

Create curls

Curling your hair doesn't have to be difficult. Try these three techniques and see which works best for you.

Use heated rollers

Take sections of nearly-dried hair. Prep with a curling spray, then wind the ends around the hot roller. Roll this under and secure it with a clip near the head. Work around the head until all your hair is rolled up. Leave in place until the rollers have cooled and the hair has set – about half an hour. Then unwind the rollers, twizzling each curl into a corkscrew.

Using a curling wand

Wind small sections of dry hair around the barrel of a curling wand. Hold for a few seconds, until the curl has set, then unwind it.

Use pin curls

Apply styling product to towel-dried hair. Working section by section, blow-dry your hair smooth using a round brush. As you finish each chunk, wind it into a curl and pin it against your head. Let the curls cool down so that they set properly, then unpin them.

1940s curls

Prep your hair with curling spray and create curls using pin curls or rollers. If you're using rollers, make sure you use big ones – smaller rollers will give you tighter curls, which might frizz up when you brush them out.

Once the curls have set, tip your head back and carefully rake your fingers through your hair, and then brush it through with a paddle brush. Most of the curls will drop down in long, smooth waves, leaving you with a Hollywood goddess look. Pull these around to one side of your neck, curl the ends with your fingers, and finish with lots of hairspray. Complete the look with red lipstick and a flick of black eyeliner.

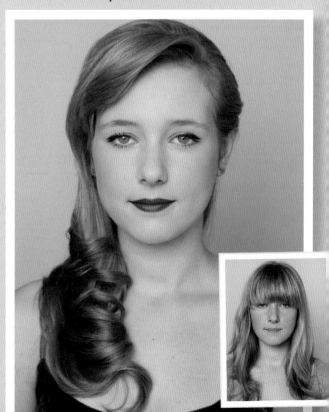

Beachy waves

The idea here is to create artfully tousled hair, so you look like you've come from a lazy day at the beach. The easiest way to make waves is with a curling wand. Rough-dry your hair, then blow-dry it until it's fairly smooth.

Taking small sections, curl each in turn until you have a head full of cooling corkscrew curls. Then ... get creative. Rake your fingers through the curls to pull them down into waves. For a real seaside effect, spritz with a salt-water spray, which will add texture and make your hair a bit sticky, and then separate the waves until you have an authentically un-styled-looking result.

Super straight

You can blow-dry your hair straight, working in sections. Hold each section of hair taut with a brush while you move the dryer down the hair from root to tip. This smoothes down the cuticle, the outer layer the hair. When the cuticle is smooth, it reflects light more evenly, which makes hair look shiny.

If you use straighteners, be careful that your hair is properly dry before you start – otherwise, the water in each hair boils, expands and damages the cuticle from the inside, making the hair more fragile. Use a heat-protective spray to stop the hair getting scorched and damaged.

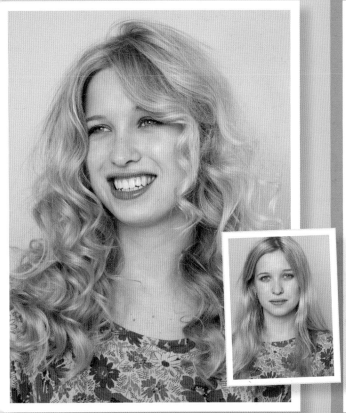

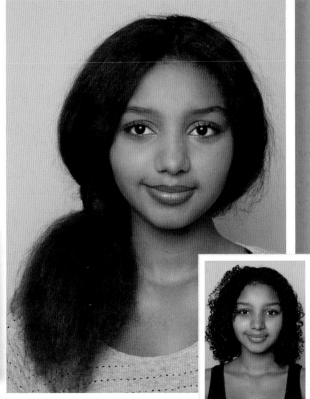

33 put your hair up

Yes, you can be the belle of the ball. Learn to create a cool "up-do" and you'll never be short of a party hairstyle. These looks are impressive but they're not impossible.

1. High ponytail

Blow-dry your hair smooth then, combing the top and sides to get it as smooth and flat as possible, pull back and secure in a high ponytail. Spray the front and sides with hairspray, and comb through to keep it all super-smooth. Take a small section of hair from underneath the "tail" and carefully wind it round the hair elastic, to hide it, and secure underneath with a grip.

2. Quiff

Towel-dry your hair, work a medium-hold styling product through it, then rough-dry it to remove most of the water. Comb your hair through and blow-dry it so that it lies flat and close to the head at the sides. At the top, you want to get as much lift as possible. Do this by pulling the brush through your hair and lifting it up to stretch the hair from the roots while you're blowdrying. Then flip the front section of hair over to one side. Use a kirby grip or a touch of gel to secure it in place, and finish with hairspray.

3. Braids

Start by practising braids on a friend, as it's easier to see what you're doing on someone else. Starting in the middle of the head, plait down one side as you would do for a French plait, taking a small section of hair from each side as you work. When you reach the nape of the neck, plait down the length of the hair, then coil up the resulting plait and pin into place. Then do the other side. Blowdrying your hair smooth before you start will give you a sleeker result.

4. Cornrows

It takes practice to get cornrows neat and even, so they might be a bit bumpy at first.

Separate out a section of hair in the line that you want the first cornrow to follow. Comb it through with conditioning spray or gel. This will keep the hair smooth, and since damp hair stretches a bit, the plaits will tighten as they dry. Take a small chunk of hair at the front of the row, divide it into three, and make the first twists in the plait. Keeping two parts of the plait out to the side, take a few of the next hairs in the row and add them into the middle of the plait. Keep the plait as close to the head as you can but don't pull the hair too tight or it will be painful.

Carry on until you reach the edge of the scalp. Then plait to the ends of the hair and secure the end of the plait with a clip or hair elastic. Plait the rest of hair into rows until you've done the whole head.

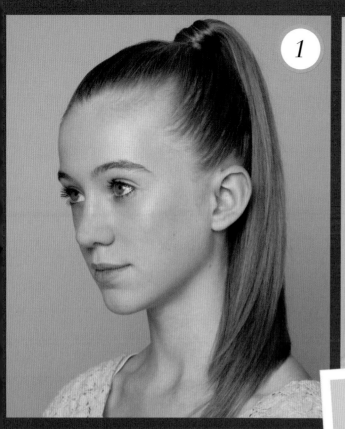

1

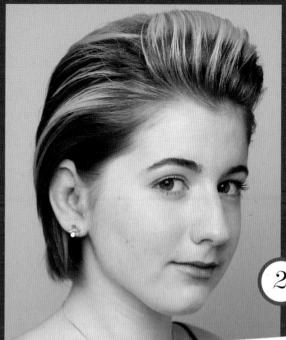

2

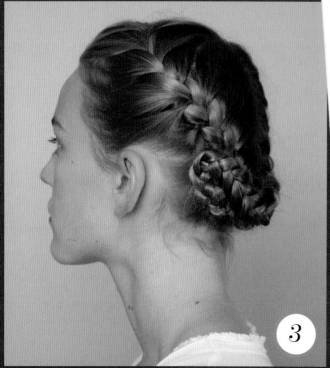

3

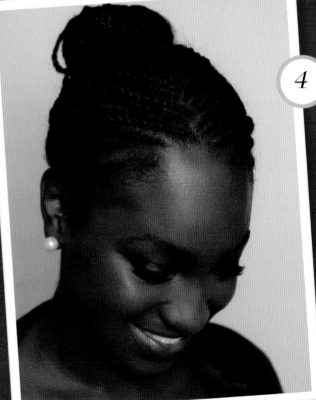

4

51

Beth's signature
hair look: the
chopstick up-do

Q Why do you like this look?
A It's simple but it looks quite impressive.

Q Does it take ages?
A No, it's really quick, but it does take a bit of practice. You have to hold your hair in a bunch and put the chopstick (or pencil) to the left of the bunch – don't push it through your hair yet. Working clockwise, wind all your hair onto the chopstick. Then up-end the whole parcel of hair and stab the chopstick back down through the coiled hair at the back, to hold it in place.

Q Any tips?
A It's easier if your hair isn't too clean and slippery.

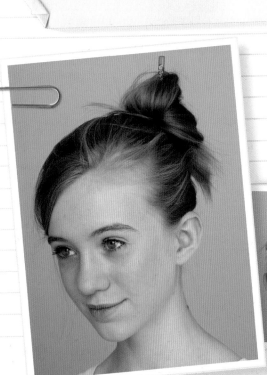

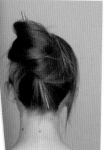

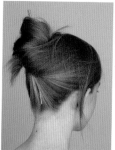

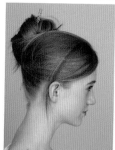

52

Nails

Your nails are like a mini canvas on which you can express yourself. Keep them plain and neat, paint them every colour of the rainbow, or decorate them with glitter and crystals. The possibilities are endless, so go play.

WHAT THE EXPERT SAYS

Nail technician Andrea Fulerton spends her working days tending to the talons of super-celebs. Here are her top tips:

☑ **Paint nail varnish on in thin coats.**
This is the best way to get it to last – thick coats are prone to chipping. Before you start, clean the nails with varnish remover to make sure there's no oil on the nail plate. Always rest your hand on a flat surface to steady it.

☑ **Say goodbye to smudges.** If your varnish smudges, dip a finger in nail varnish remover and swipe over the smudged surface to help merge the smudge back in. If you're in a rush when doing your nails, stick to neutral colours. They don't show smudges and dents half as much as bright colours.

☑ **Prevent hang nails.** These are rough spikes of skin which appear when the skin at the edge of your nails becomes dry and cracked. Using hand cream and nail oil keeps hands moisturized and helps prevent them. If you do get a hang nail, snip it off very carefully using cuticle trimmers.

34 strengthen your nails

There are lots of small things you can do that will make a big difference to your nails.

❤ Make sure you're eating enough protein. Nails, like hair, are made of protein.

❤ Use special strengthening products that you paint onto your nails. These will sink in and help your nails harden up.

❤ If you have ridges in your nails, it may be because you are short of B vitamins. The quickest way to boost your vitamin B levels is to take a vitamin supplement, but for all-round health, it's really worth making sure that you're eating a balanced diet (see pages 115–123).

❤ If you break a nail, gently lever your nail clippers under the broken edge and snip it off, then gently file the jagged edge smooth. File all your nails down to one length – if you don't, you'll always have different length nails. This way, at least you'll have groomed, uniform nails.

tip Soaking your nails in water really softens them up, so when you need to cut your toenails or fingernails, do it straight after a bath or shower.

35 get rid of white nail spots

Lots of people think that when you see little white spots in your nails, it's because you aren't eating enough calcium, but you're more likely to have a mild zinc deficiency. It's easy to correct this by taking zinc supplements. You should stop getting white spots within a few weeks.

36 help your nails grow

Massaging oil into your cuticles every night nourishes the nail bed (the bit the nail grows from) and stimulates circulation, which helps the bit of the nail beneath the surface that is actively growing. Cuticle oil is specially designed to be easily absorbed, but you could use any oil, such as almond or olive oil, though it may leave your hands a bit stickier. If you bite your nails or skin, try giving up one finger at a time. Once you see the improvement in the fingers you've left alone, you may give up biting the others, too.

37 think of your nails as jewels, not tools

Using your nails to scrape stickers off books or prise things open is asking for trouble. If your nails are on the weak side, it will make them split and break. Look after them!

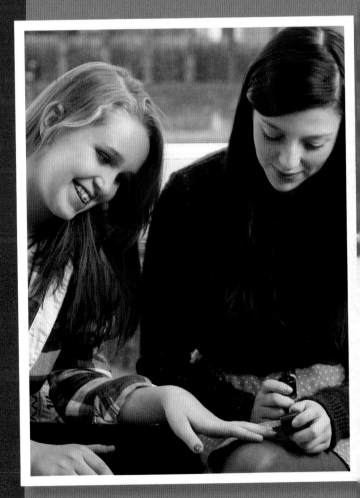

38 give yourself a manicure and pedicure

It's not difficult. Give yourself a bit of time, line up everything you need before you start, and enjoy yourself.

You will need:

- ♥ A bowl of hot water
- ♥ Varnish remover
- ♥ Cotton wool
- ♥ Nail scissors (nail clippers for toes)
- ♥ Nail file
- ♥ Cuticle cream (optional)
- ♥ Cuticle stick
- ♥ Hand cream
- ♥ Toe separators (or two tissues) for keeping toes apart
- ♥ Nail varnish, plus base coat and top coat (clear varnish will do if you don't have special ones)

Step-by-step manicure and pedicure

1. Remove any old nail varnish, then trim your nails and file them smooth (don't file your toenails down too much at the sides, because it can encourage them to become ingrown).

2. If you're using cuticle cream, rub it into the nail beds and then soak your hands or feet in hot water for a few minutes. This will help the cream to soften up the cuticles.

3. Ease back the cuticles with a cuticle stick. Then wash off the cuticle cream and wipe the nails with varnish remover to prepare the nail surface for painting.

4. Paint on a layer of base coat. This helps the varnish to stay on better, and it stops the varnish staining your nails.

5. Paint on a layer of varnish. Let it dry, then paint on another, and let this dry too.

6. Paint on a layer of clear top coat. It makes the varnish super-shiny and makes it last longer, too.

tip You can paint layers of varnish on one after another, which is what would happen in a beauty salon, but it will take hours to dry properly and harden up – so if you're doing a pedicure, get your flip-flops out.

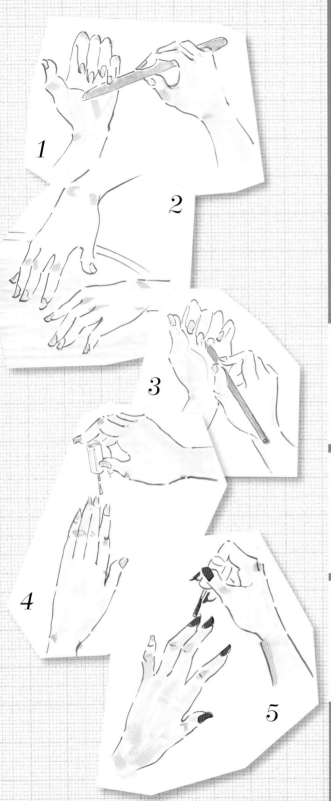

1

2

3

4

5

39 wrap your nails

This is the easiest way to get complex designs onto your nails. Applying the wraps is a bit fiddly and you need to be careful not to knock up the edges once they're on … but it's well worth it for the wow factor. Here are some nail wrap looks from Nail Rock.

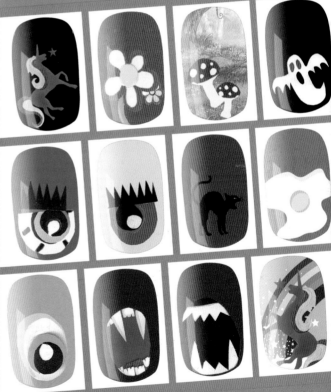

Nails

40 **try your hand at nail design**

Make your nails stand out with these eye-catching looks from WAH Nails, a top London nail salon. You'll need a few nail art pens in different colours.

1. 60s chic: use the same colours (pink base with black and white stripes) but vary the design on each nail.

2. Melted ice cream: start with a yellow under-layer, then paint on pink as if it's been dribbled over the top.

3. Doodles and squiggles: layer on varied base colours, then let your imagination – and squiggles – run riot.

4. Space age: paint geometric patterns in black over a base of blue.

5. Electric crackle: paint horizontal stripes across your nails in contrasting colours. When they've dried, paint a layer of black shatter nail polish over the top. This will crack, revealing the colours underneath.

6. Aztec bright: on a base of yellow, add stripes of contrasting colour, then paint on black detailing and white spots.

7. Candy stripes: paint each nail a different colour, then top with white stripes.

8. Leopard print: choose your base colour, then add blobs of white and edge them in black.

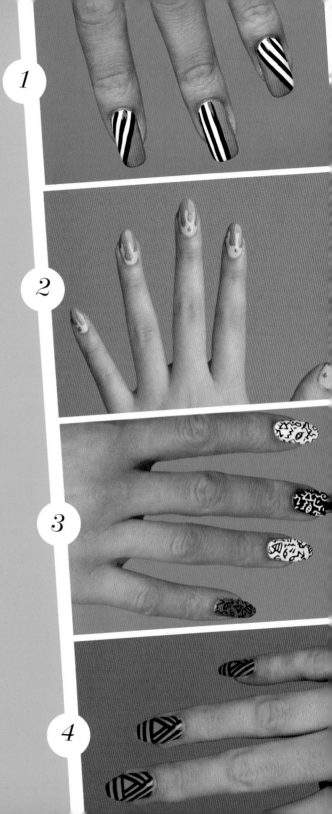

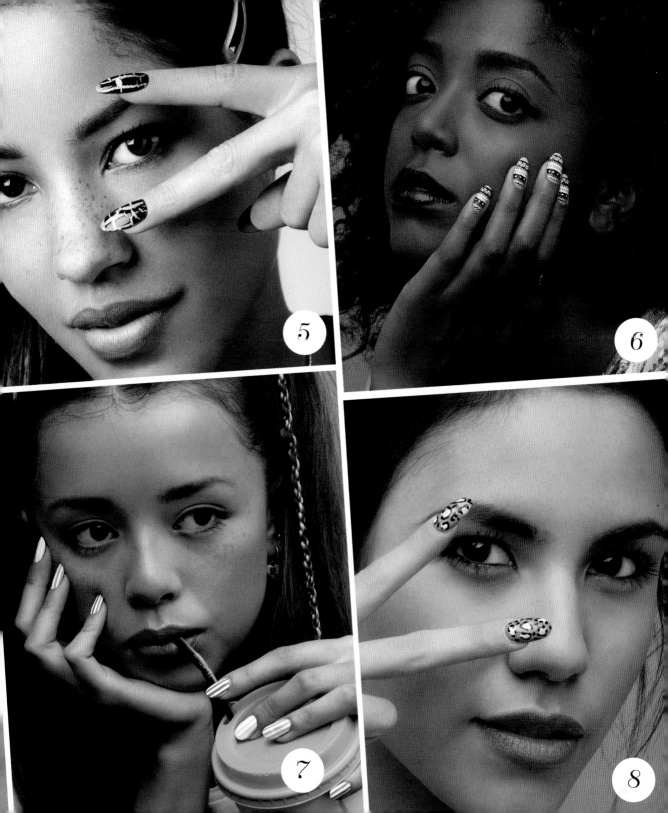

Beth gets creative with her nails

Q How do you like to decorate your nails?

A Normally I just paint my nails one colour, but sometimes I try making them more interesting by painting patterns on my nails with different colours. Nail tattoos are fun, too.

Q Aren't they really tricky to use?

A Not really. They're pretty small so they're a bit fiddly to apply, but they have sticky backs so all you have to do is put them in place and use a top coat to fix them.

Q So what have we here?

A These are leopard-print nails, done with a really fine-tipped nail art pen on a turquoise base. On the little fingers, the "spots" are filled in with fluoro-pink varnish.

Q Did you paint them yourself?

A No. But now I know how to do it, I can't wait to try it myself.

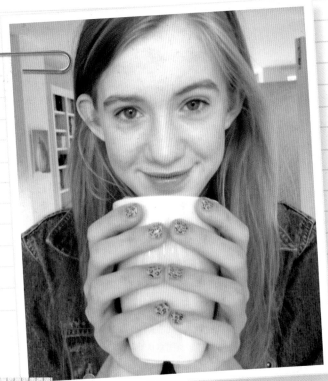

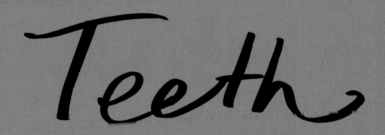

Teeth

Want your teeth to be strong, white
and healthy? Want them to last a lifetime?
All you have to do is put in a bit of effort
every day to keep them clean, fresh and
looking their best.

41 brush your teeth properly

You've been told to a million times but, seriously, it is well worth getting into the habit of brushing your teeth properly. This is why:

For health
♥ Proper brushing (and flossing) removes plaque from your teeth.

♥ It helps keep your gums healthy and prevents gum disease.

♥ It reduces your chances of getting decay and cavities in your teeth.

For vanity
♥ Thorough brushing keeps your teeth as white as possible by getting rid of stains on the surface of your teeth.

♥ It keeps your breath fresh – particularly if you always brush your tongue as well as your teeth.

Why plaque is bad news for teeth
You can't see it, but plaque coats your teeth with a sticky film of bacteria. When you eat something sweet, these bacteria make the plaque acidic. Then the plaque eats into the enamel of your teeth and begins to wear it away – and this is where decay can set in. Get rid of the plaque and your teeth will be much healthier.

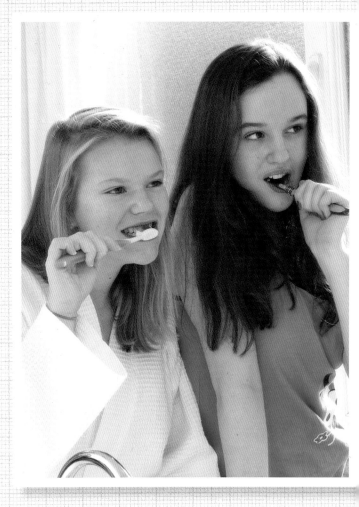

What is "thorough brushing"?
♦ Spending two minutes carefully working around your mouth, tooth by tooth.

♦ Brushing the insides of your teeth as carefully as the outsides.

♦ Concentrating on the bit where the tooth joins the gum.

♦ Using an electric toothbrush.

42 start power brushing

Invest in an electric toothbrush. It's like the difference between using a washing machine to clean your clothes and washing them by hand. Both will get your clothes clean but the machine will do it much more quickly and thoroughly. Studies have shown that you remove twice as much plaque with an electric brush as with a manual toothbrush in the same time.

tip Spit, don't rinse. Today's high-tech toothpastes are full of ingredients which are really good for teeth – they cut down on bacteria levels and protect your teeth with a layer of fluoride. So once you've used this wonderful stuff on your teeth, don't rinse it away. Spit out the excess and leave the rest in your mouth to do its work.

43 wear a mouthguard when you play sport

Ask your parents to invest in a proper mouthguard if you do any contact sports. Your teeth will love you for it.

WHAT THE EXPERT SAYS

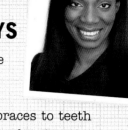

Dr Uchenna Okoye is a dentist who specializes in everything from braces to teeth whitening. Here are her top tips:

☑ **Think prevention rather than cure.**
If your gums bleed, it's a sign that you have gum disease and you need to brush your teeth more, not less. Work on the basics, brushing twice a day, using floss daily and seeing your hygienist regularly.

☑ **Recharge your teeth with fluoride.**
Fluoride makes teeth more resistant to attack by plaque bacteria. For maximum effect use a fluoride toothpaste and rinse with a fluoride mouthwash every day.

☑ **Protect your teeth from acid attack.**
Don't brush your teeth straight after eating sweets or drinking juice. These things make your mouth acidic, and brushing rubs in the acidity and wears your enamel away. Instead, rinse with water and follow with mouthwash.

☑ **Think twice before whitening.**
Teenagers can have their teeth whitened, but it's vital the treatment is carried out by an experienced dentist. Whitening can make teeth very sensitive, and this side effect is worse the younger you are. It's best to wait until you're seventeen.

44 floss, floss, floss!

Flossing is the best way to remove plaque and debris from between your teeth and keep your mouth clean. It's also one of the best ways of preventing bad breath (just smell the floss after it's been used).

How to floss

❤ Make sure you are sliding the floss under the gums, to help shift plaque below the gum line.

❤ Get a good grip on the floss and curl it around each tooth for maximum effect.

45 wash your mouth out

Use mouthwash when you haven't brushed (if you use it straight after brushing it will rinse off the helpful ingredients in toothpaste).

Why mouthwash is worth using

❤ It keeps your breath fresh.

❤ It keeps levels of bacteria down, so it reduces plaque.

❤ A fluoride mouthwash will help protect your teeth.

tip If you really don't like using floss, try inter-dental sticks – tiny spiral brushes on a flexible wire – which you can poke into the gaps between teeth to clean them out.

46 embrace braces

Yes, it's a pain to have your smile spoiled by train-track braces for a year or two, and yes, it will pinch every time they're tightened, but braces are still the best way to realign your teeth, and your teens are the ideal time to do this.

So, if your dentist thinks that you might benefit from braces, go with it. You won't regret it. Dr Uchenna Okoye says, "I have a huge number of adult patients who come to me for orthodontic treatment to straighten out their teeth. Even though they may be in their thirties or forties, they're still cross with their parents for not sorting out their teeth when they were younger."

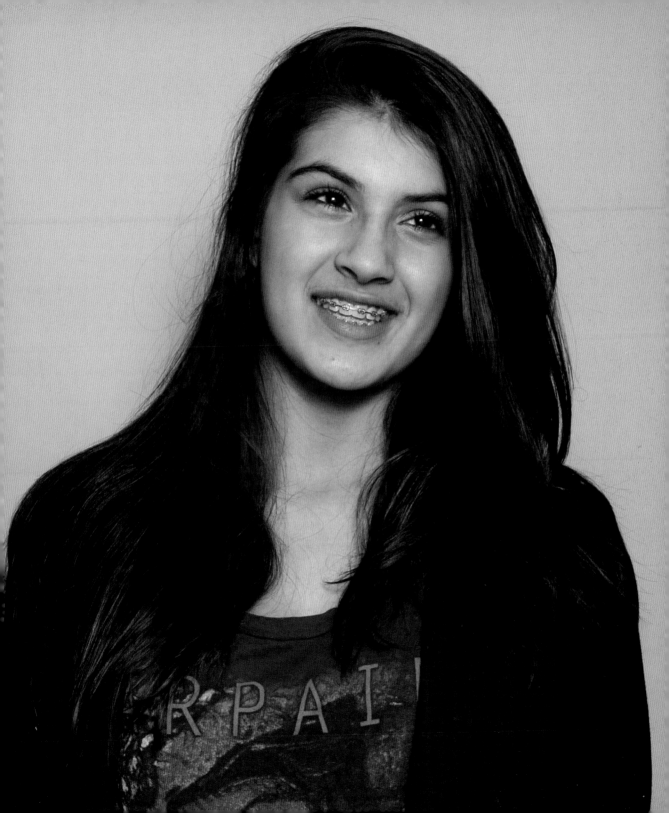

How Beth felt about her braces

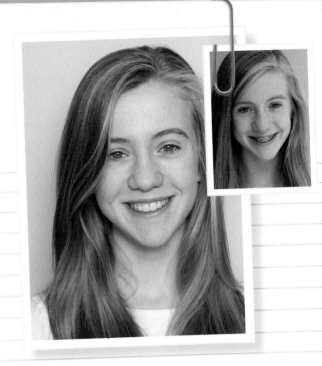

Q Why did you need braces?

A My teeth weren't bad but they were what the orthodontist called "untidy". Some of them were crowded together and some of them overlapped the ones next to them. That meant I needed braces on my upper and lower teeth for about fifteen months.

Q How did you feel about having to wear them?

A I didn't mind too much because lots of my friends had train-track braces at the same time, and I knew they would improve my teeth. It was annoying not being able to eat whatever I wanted — I couldn't eat things like nuts or chewing gum at all.

Q What's the worst thing about braces?

A When they put a stronger wire along the brackets, it really aches, so you may need painkillers. Tell your parents to be sympathetic and give you food that doesn't need much chewing, such as soup or mashed potato.

Q Was it worth it?

A Definitely! I can see the difference and I like my smile more now. I have a retainer which I need to wear all the time for another year, but that's easy.

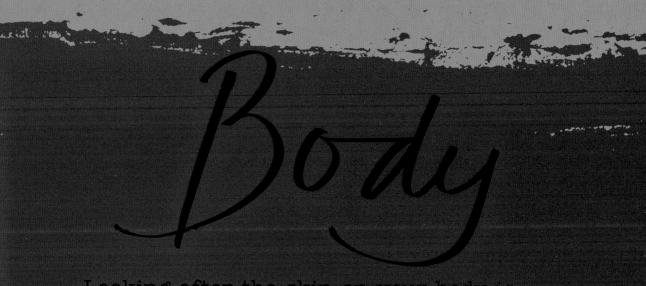

Body

Looking after the skin on your body is as important as looking after the skin on your face. The basics are exactly the same – just cleanse, exfoliate and moisturize.

WHAT THE EXPERT SAYS

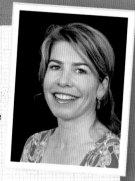

Dr Jennifer Jones is a dermatologist at the Royal Free Hospital in London. Here are her top tips:

☑ **Moisturize all over every day.** If you have sensitive skin, choose an unfragranced moisturizer. If you often have very dry or inflamed red skin, consult your GP as you may have a common skin disease such as eczema or psoriasis. These can usually be treated effectively with prescription creams.

☑ **Check your moles.** It's very important to start checking your moles in your teens. Take a photo of them so you know what you're starting with. Look out for any mole which stands out from the others. Dermatologists call this the "ugly duckling sign". Look for any new moles, and remember the "ABCDE" signs – Asymmetry, irregular Borders, more than two Colours (especially reds and blacks), increasing Diameter, Evolution (change). If you see these, see a doctor.

☑ **Don't just wear sunscreen on your face.** In the summer, wear sunscreen on any skin that's exposed to the sun. Get into the habit of carrying sunscreen in your bag, so you can reapply it if you're outdoors for a while.

47 have a shower or bath every day

During the day your body perspires, even when you don't realize it, and puberty makes your sweat glands more active, too.

The sweat glands all over your body produce a watery sweat that doesn't smell much, but the glands in your armpits and groin produce a smellier kind of sweat. They react when you're nervous as well as when you're hot. When that second kind of sweat gets trapped in your armpits and reacts with the bacteria on your skin, you start to smell – so wash it all off every day.

tip Dr Jennifer Jones says: if you have rough red skin on your upper arms or thighs this may be a common skin condition called keratosis pilaris. The best way to treat it is with moisturizers containing urea. If the skin gets inflamed, see a doctor.

48 wear deodorant

Use an anti-perspirant deodorant. It will cover up the smell of sweat, and also reduce the amount of sweat your body produces, so you'll always smell fresh.

49 get into body brushing

Brushing yourself all over with a stiff-bristled body brush is a great way to remove dead skin. It improves lymph drainage so it's good for your health, too.

How to brush your body

Your skin needs to be completely dry before you brush your body.

1. Using gentle strokes, start at your feet and work up to your knees, then your thighs. Work all around your legs, covering every bit of skin.

2. Brush your arms, starting with the wrists and working up towards your neck. If you can reach it, brush your back, too.

3. Finish off by brushing in a circular motion around your tummy.

69

Body

50 get smooth

When you want to deal with body hair should you shave it off? Or rip it out? This is what you need to know about the different ways to be hair free.

How to use	Pros
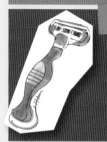 **Razors** In the shower, lather up with shaving gel, shower gel or conditioner, to help the razor glide smoothly. Then gently slide the razor up your legs, against the direction the hairs are growing in.	Shaving is quick and cheap, and you can do it whenever you like. Don't believe anyone who says shaving makes your hair grow back thicker and darker – it doesn't!
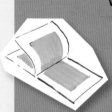 **Waxing** You can wax your own legs, or get them waxed in a salon. In a salon, wax is smoothed onto your legs. Then a cotton strip is pressed onto the wax and whisked away, taking the hair with it.	After waxing, your skin will be beautifully smooth, and the hair will take weeks to grow back.
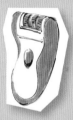 **Epilation** Epilators are handheld electrical devices with whirling blades that pull hairs out at the roots. Hold your skin taut, and slide the epilator up your leg as you would with a razor.	If you are thorough, you can get very good results. Because epilators can grab very short hairs you can deal with regrowth as soon as it appears.
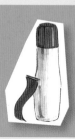 **Creams** Hair-removal creams, gels and mousses need to be left on the skin for a few minutes while they dissolve the keratin in the hair, so it comes loose from its follicles. Then you can scrape the hair away.	Because they remove hair from just below the skin's surface, the results last longer than shaving. They're very easy to use, too.

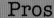

70

Cons

You'll need to change your razor regularly (a blunt blade isn't much use). Shaving doesn't last long, and your hair will grow back stubbly.

The first time you try waxing, the pain may take you by surprise. Your skin may be a little sore and red after you wax. Be careful if you wax at home – you can end up bruising your legs.

Epilating hurts, especially the first time you try it. It's best to stick to your arms and legs – areas such as the armpits, bikini line and face are much trickier and are sensitive.

Hair-removal creams usually smell horrible. They contain chemicals, so do a patch test: use the cream on a small patch of skin, 24 hours before you use it for real, in case you have an allergic reaction to it.

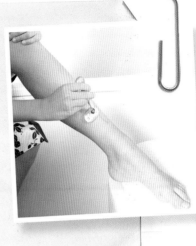

Beth on shaving

Q How do you feel about hair removal?
A So far, all I've tried is shaving.

Q How did you find that?
A It's pretty easy as long as you have a good razor and plenty of time. If you have a razor with built in gel strips on it, then you don't even need to use shaving foam or gel.

Q Any tips?
A Don't shave in too much of a hurry – you might miss bits or you might cut yourself.

Q What about waxing?
A I feel that waxing would be better than shaving because it removes hair from the root and lasts much longer. I'd like to try it but I've been told it's really painful. But I like the idea of waxing much more than epilating. That sounds like torture and slow, too. At least waxing is quick!

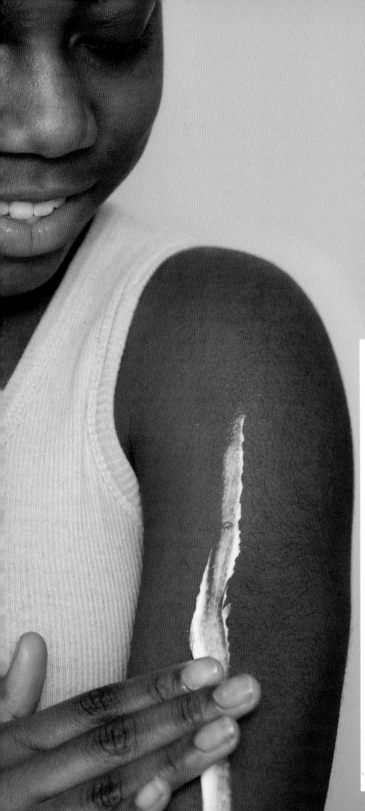

51 exfoliate and moisturize

The top layer of your skin is constantly shedding itself – in fact, most household dust is made up of dead skin. Using a body scrub or an exfoliating wash cloth once or twice a week helps lift away dead cells and leave your skin smoother and fresher. If your skin feels dry after exfoliating, use a body moisturizer to keep it feeling soft.

Make your own body scrub

Put two tablespoons of sugar in a small bowl. Stir in enough oil (olive oil, sweet almond oil, jojoba oil, whatever you have to hand) to make a paste. Now you have a scrub which you can use in the shower. Rub it into damp skin, then rinse off. For a stronger exfoliating effect, use it on dry skin before you start showering.

Variations

❤ Use sea salt instead of sugar, or mix sea salt and sugar together. Salt crystals are sharper than sugar so it will feel rougher on your skin.

❤ Add oatmeal to the scrub. Oats contain proteins which are soothing to the skin.

❤ Add a drop of essential oil such as lavender or rose oil to the mixing oil, to make the scrub smell amazing.

52 give a friend a massage

Massage is a great way to relax tired, tight muscles. You don't need professional training to make it soothing and effective. Just work slowly, and use smooth but firm movements. Pressing on any knotty bits of muscle for twenty seconds will make the knots soften – but don't press too hard unless you're asked to.

Shoulder massage

1. Start with your fingers resting on the top of your friend's shoulders and use your thumbs to work into the muscles on either side of the spine. Work outwards first, and then down both sides.

2. Gently pinch the whole muscle at the top of the shoulders.

3. Using your knuckles, lightly sweep down the muscles at the sides of the neck, from the ear to the shoulder.

Foot massage

1. Massage the feet with firm, strong movements (if you're too gentle, it really tickles). Massage the top of the feet, around the ankles, the back of the heels and the soles of the feet, too.

2. Work down the top of the foot. Do this with the foot pointing towards you, your thumbs on top of the foot and your fingers underneath. Run your thumbs down in between the bones on the foot, sweeping down towards the gaps between the toes.

3. Massage up and down the underside of the foot. Use your thumbs to work into the ball of the foot, using little circular movements, or make your knuckles into a fist and carefully work that across the ball and down the middle of the foot.

4. Massage each toe, pulling gently from where it joins the foot to the tip.

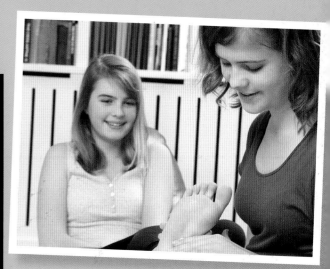

Four massage movements

♦ Long, sweeping movements using the heels of your hands.

♦ Muscle-loosening work with your thumbs.

♦ Gently squeezing muscles between your fingers and thumbs.

♦ Light friction, rubbing your palms back and forth, flat against the skin.

53 learn the basics of body language

The way you act can really give away how you're feeling. When you're face-to-face with another person, experts reckon that as little as ten per cent of what you communicate comes from the words you say. At least half of what other people pick up comes from your body language, and the rest from your tone of voice. So what's your body saying?

Good stuff

A genuine smile: you look friendly, happy and approachable. It needs to be a real smile – one that uses all of your face, not just your mouth.

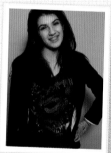

Tilting your head or framing your face with your hands: it looks like you're really listening to the other person – though it also draws attention to yourself.

"Mirroring" the other person's movements: it sounds odd, but most of us do this automatically when we're with people we like. We sit or stand in the same way, lean on our elbows when they're doing it, take a sip

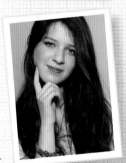

of our drink when they take one of theirs. It's normal behaviour and it puts people at ease by making them feel that you like them, trust them and agree with them.

Having a relaxed, easy stance: you look approachable, confident and at ease.

Making proper eye contact: you look interested and as if you're paying attention. People who refuse to make eye contact seem nervous and shifty, or could be lying.

Bad stuff

Folded arms: you look cross, especially if you stick your chin out defiantly at the same time. This is the clearest sign possible that you're putting up a barrier between you and anyone you're with. You may as well be wearing a big sign saying, "Stay away!"

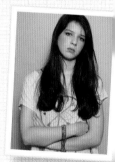

Ducking your head, slouching, or shrinking down in your chair: you look shy, or as if you wish you weren't there.

Biting your lip or touching your face: you look anxious or uncomfortable. Biting your nails or picking at your clothes also makes you look nervous.

Standing with one leg (or worse, both) pointing towards the door: it looks as if you want to make a quick getaway.

Pointing your finger at someone: you could look like you're asserting yourself, but more often it just looks aggressive.

Clothes

What you wear makes a huge statement about who you are and how you feel about life. So where do you start and what do you choose? Here's how to get it right and look fabulous every day.

54 dress to flatter your body shape

The shape of your body affects the way you look in clothes. That might seem blindingly obvious, but if you have a rough idea of what shape you are, it's easier to work out what clothes will suit you.

Bear in mind that the body types opposite are very generalized. You may not be completely one shape or another. Also, remember that the kind of clothes that suit you will depend on your character as well as your body shape, so these are suggestions, not rules. You might tick all the right boxes for wearing, say, a puff-sleeved, flower-print dress, but if it feels all wrong when you put it on, go with your instincts and choose something else. If you feel good in what you're wearing, the chances are you'll look good.

Shape

Pear

Wider at the hips than the shoulders.

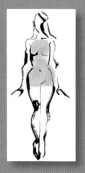

Athletic

Wider at the shoulders than the hips.

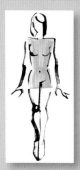

Hourglass

Curvy, with a small waist.

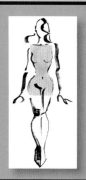

Boyish

Straight up and down and flat-chested.

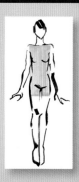

What to wear	What to avoid
Anything that boosts the proportions of your top half and streamlines your lower half. That could be chunky jumpers, jackets or tops with structured, padded or puffed shoulders, or empire-line tops and dresses. To keep your hips and legs looking sleek, try close-fitting skirts (minis, pencil skirts and maxis can all look good) and neat narrow or boot-cut jeans.	Pleat-front trousers and A-line or kilted skirts, which add volume to your hips, and close-fitting cropped cardigans which will shrink your top half while emphasizing your bottom.
Outfits that balance out your top and bottom halves. Look for tops that are a sleek fit, to show off your shoulders without making them look any bigger than they already are (halter necks are great in summer). Try pairing neat jackets or cardigans with A-line skirts, flared trousers, boyfriend jeans or harem pants. If you're tall, maxi dresses may work for you.	Padded shoulders which can turn you into a top-heavy triangle. Frilly shirts and dresses and double-breasted coats and jackets won't do you many favours, either.
Figure-friendly clothes that define your waist and skim your curves. Wrap dresses and cardigans will probably suit you, as will belted dresses or coats, and fitted jeans that aren't too low on the hips. If you have a big bust, choose scoop-necked tops (ones with a deeper, curvier neckline) rather than round-necked tops (like a traditional man's T-shirt) or high-necked tops (like a roll-neck).	High-necked or round-necked tops, ribbed polo-necks, loose tops and bulky jumpers (these will make you look solid from shoulders to hips). If you have short legs, avoid cropped trousers or leggings – these will make your legs looks shorter.
Clothes where you can play with proportion – because you can get away with it. Look out for tops with a high neckline or a roll neck, peasant blouses, ruched tops and dresses. Experiment with stripes and bold prints, oversized jumpers and T-shirts, mini skirts and maxi dresses, cropped trousers, flares and skinny jeans.	Short, clingy dresses (you'll look skinny, but that's about it), and baggy boyfriend trousers (they'll only make you look more boyish).

Clothes

55 find your personal style

Trends are half the fun of fashion, but just because everyone else is wearing dayglo legwarmers, that doesn't mean you have to. Try to work out what your own personal style is — the kind of clothes you look great and feel comfortable in — and tip the trend in your own direction rather than following it slavishly.

56 value vintage

Once, old clothes were just ... old clothes. But now, anything more than a few years old is hailed as "vintage". Recycling clothes like this is eco-friendly, inexpensive and provides you with something unique that no one else will have, so plunge in at your local charity shop and have a rummage.

tip Find someone that knows you well — your best friend, sister or mum — and ask them what styles they think suit you best.

57 play up your best points

It's crucial to think positively about your body shape. We can all find something about ourselves we don't like – even gorgeous models have bits of their bodies they say they hate – but focus on the things you do like instead. Choose clothes that emphasize the great bits of your body and you'll look and feel fantastic.

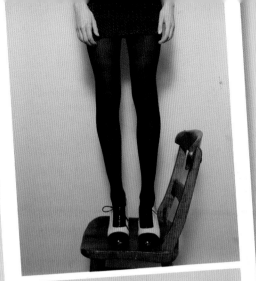

Draw attention to your strong points

❤ If you have slim legs, show them off in skinny jeans or short skirts.

❤ If you like your arms, wear sleeveless tops in summer or skinny jumpers in winter.

❤ If you have a curvy figure, go for dresses or coats that are belted at the waist.

❤ If you have a small chest, try high-necked jumpers and double-breasted jackets.

❤ If you have gorgeous ankles, put them on display with cropped trousers.

❤ If you have an elegant neck, choose a top with a modest neckline and pile your hair up like a ballerina, to show it off.

❤ If you have a small waist, flaunt it with a belt.

❤ If you have a big bust try closely-fitted scoop-neck tops.

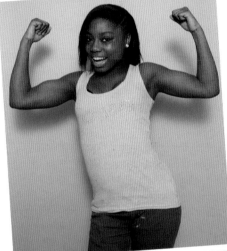

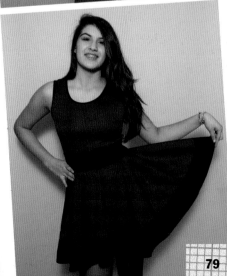

58 work out which colours suit you

You can wear any colours you like, but you may have noticed that some colours suit you better than others. Find the right ones and they'll make you look lively and well. You'll know the wrong ones because they'll make you look tired and drab.

Work out what looks best

Professional colour analysts will find colours that suit you by draping you in a succession of scarves of different colours. You can try a version of this at home.

1. Get together with your friends and ask everyone to bring as many different brightly coloured clothes or scarves as they can, so that you have a good variety between you.

2. Take it in turns to hold the different colours up near your face (drape them over your shoulder, or wear them like a scarf). Ask your friends to decide whether it's a good or bad shade for you. It's good to get other people's opinions on this because they'll often make you try a colour that you'd never have dreamed of wearing, and it might just be the right one for you.

Colour tips

❤ White shirts are quite harsh because they can make your eyes and teeth look dull by comparison. Cream tops or shirts are more flattering as they're kinder on the complexion and make your eyes and teeth look whiter.

❤ Yellow and orange tend to look awful on pale skin, but look brilliant on darker skin.

❤ There's a shade of red to suit everyone – it could be an orangey-red or a bluey-red, but you'll need to experiment to find which is right for you.

❤ People often call beige a "classic" colour. It is, but it can make pale faces look unwell.

❤ Vibrant colours like emerald green and cobalt blue are surprisingly wearable.

❤ Black can look tough, cool, chic, indie … and can also drain all the colour from your face.

❤ Dayglo colours are fun but exhausting to look at. Wear in small doses.

tip You don't have to wear bright colours head to toe. Try adding one brightly coloured item to your outfit – or even a very bright bag or scarf.

Beth goes bright

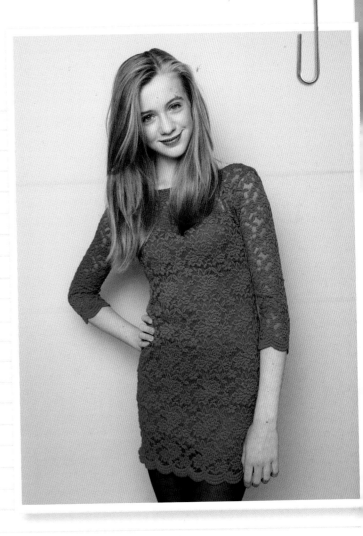

Q **Have you always been keen on colourful clothes?**

A No. I went through a phase of just wearing black and white because I thought colours didn't suit me, and that black and white looked more sophisticated.

Q **So what changed?**

A Someone said to me, "You always wear black and white," and it made me think I really should try something different. So when I went out shopping, I tried on clothes in really bright colours which I would have shied away from before.

Q **Is this blue your favourite colour?**

A One of them. I also really like bright red…

Q **What do you like about this colour?**

A It's bright and punchy and makes me feel positive and confident. I love this dress because it's an attention-grabbing colour but the shape is quite demure.

Clothes

59 discover the power of accessories

The right belt, bag, necklace – or even glasses – can make a good outfit great.

Glasses

Heavy-framed glasses add a touch of geek chic. To make glasses look more chic and less geek, make an effort with your hair, and add lipstick or lip gloss.

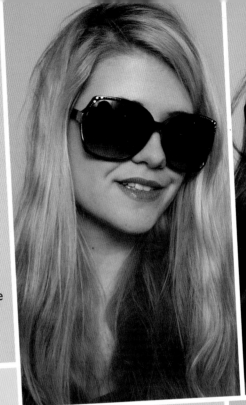

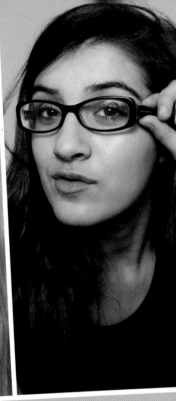

Statement jewellery

One oversized bangle, necklace or pair of earrings can become a focal point of your whole look. It doesn't have to be expensive and it can liven up the plainest outfit.

tip If you want to have your ears pierced and you're under sixteen, you'll need to take a parent or guardian with you. Reliable shops will refuse to pierce your ears otherwise. After you've had your ears pierced, follow the aftercare instructions carefully while they heal.

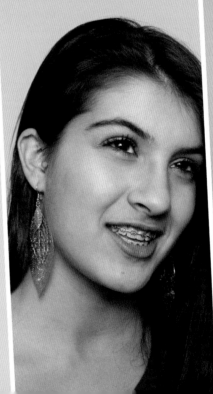

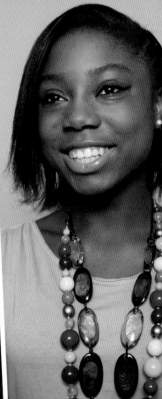

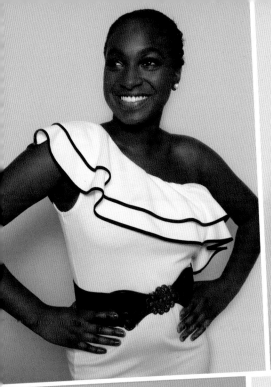

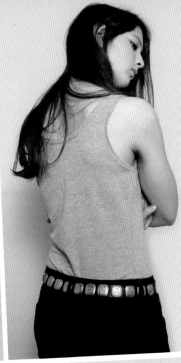

Belts

Apart from holding up your trousers, belts can cinch in a baggy shirt, cardigan, dress or coat. Charity shops and vintage stores are great places to find interesting belts. Wide belts? Skinny belts? Play around and see what suits you.

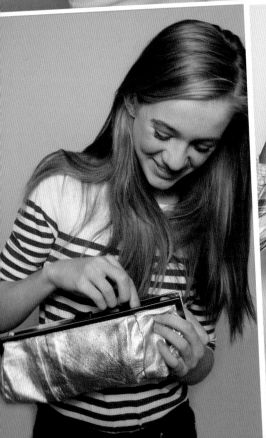

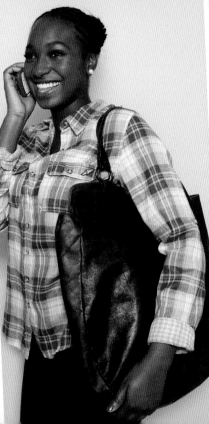

Bags

Your bag can say a lot about you, and completely change the look of your outfit. Slouchy shoulder bags give you a laid-back look, while structured handbags with handles look elegant and ladylike. Dainty purses are great for parties, but you can't fit much in them. Canvas or cotton totes can be stylish and eco-conscious at the same time – if you carry them when you go shopping, you won't have to use plastic bags.

60 wear a hat with style

Wearing a hat takes a bit of nerve – people are always going to notice, and look at you – but hats make a terrific style statement. They also keep your head warm in winter and shade your face in summer. What's not to like? Here's what different hats can say about you.

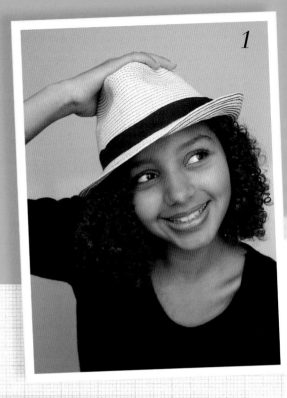

1

1. **A trilby:** tilt it back on your head and it's cheeky. Tilt it forward and it's celebrity in disguise.

2. **A tuque:** chilled out and adventurous.

3. **A trapper hat:** wild at heart.

4. **An updated cloche:** quirky and cute.

5. **A beret:** Parisian bohemian.

6. **A beanie:** laid-back and indie.

Wear with care
♦ Baseball caps – they're useful, but hard to make stylish.

♦ Outrageous or fantastical creations – unless you're channelling Lady Gaga.

♦ Fascinators – unless you're at a smart wedding.

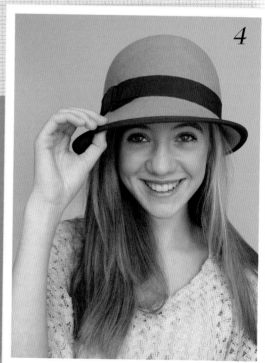

4

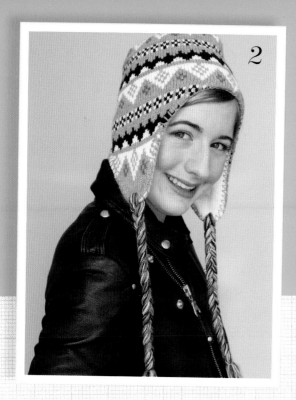

2

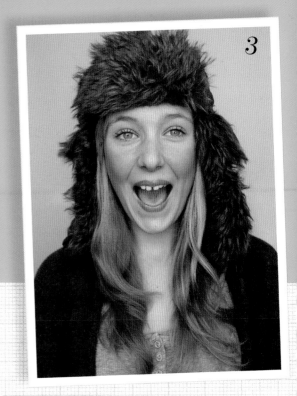

3

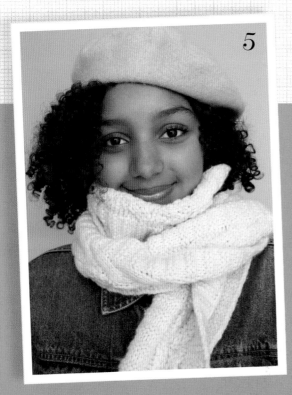

5

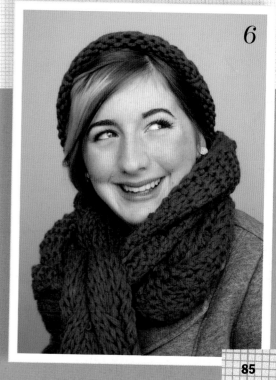

6

61 just add a scarf

Scarves aren't just for keeping you warm on a winter's day. Get creative and see what you can twist up with yours.

Wrap up in a huge scarf for **instant chic**.

Tie a scarf in a bow around your neck for a **retro look**.

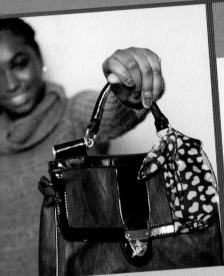
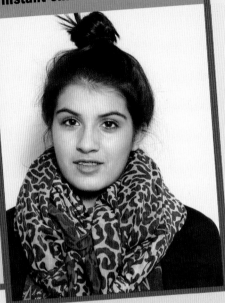
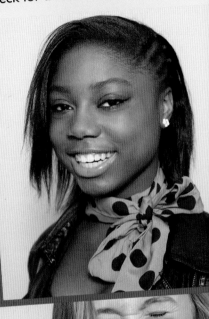

Give an ordinary-looking bag some **personality** with a bright silk scarf.

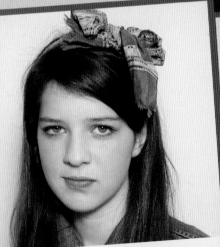
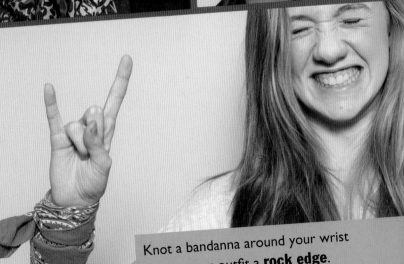

Tie a long scarf in a bow on top of your head to give your look an **indie twist**.

Knot a bandanna around your wrist to give your outfit a **rock edge**.

Exercise

Our bodies were designed to move, but we spend most of our time sitting behind desks or slumped on sofas. It doesn't take a rocket scientist to see that's not good for us. Do your body a favour and do some exercise.

WHAT THE EXPERT SAYS

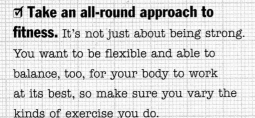

Kathryn Freeland is a personal trainer who has trained more than a few celebs. She hated exercise at school but now adores it. She devised all the exercises and routines in this chapter. Here are her top tips:

☑ **Take an all-round approach to fitness.** It's not just about being strong. You want to be flexible and able to balance, too, for your body to work at its best, so make sure you vary the kinds of exercise you do.

☑ **Exercise outside if you can.** Getting out into the fresh air is good for the soul as well as the body.

☑ **Don't worry if you don't like school exercise.** It doesn't matter if you always come last in the 100 metres or have a terror of team sports. There are lots of other ways to get moving.

☑ **Try new types of exercise.** Wall-climbing, rollerblading, dancing, ice-skating ... they're all great forms of exercise.

☑ **Get into the habit of exercising.** Then it won't be such a big deal – it will just be something you do every day.

62 find exercise that you enjoy

Exercise should be a normal part of your life. Find a kind of exercise that you actually like doing and you'll want to do it more often. Exercise can be fun, a bit of light relief from the stress of school work. The most important thing is not to put yourself off exercise for life by forcing yourself to do something that you hate.

Exercise...

❤ Keeps your body in good shape.

❤ Keeps your heart healthy.

❤ Strengthens your muscles.

❤ Improves your posture.

❤ Is sociable, if you choose a team game.

❤ Keeps your mind sharp.

❤ Helps you sleep better.

❤ Helps keep you motivated.

❤ Keeps you slim, lean and strong.

❤ Makes your body release endorphins – natural "feel-good" chemicals.

❤ Gets rid of stress by using up the adrenaline that makes you feel antsy.

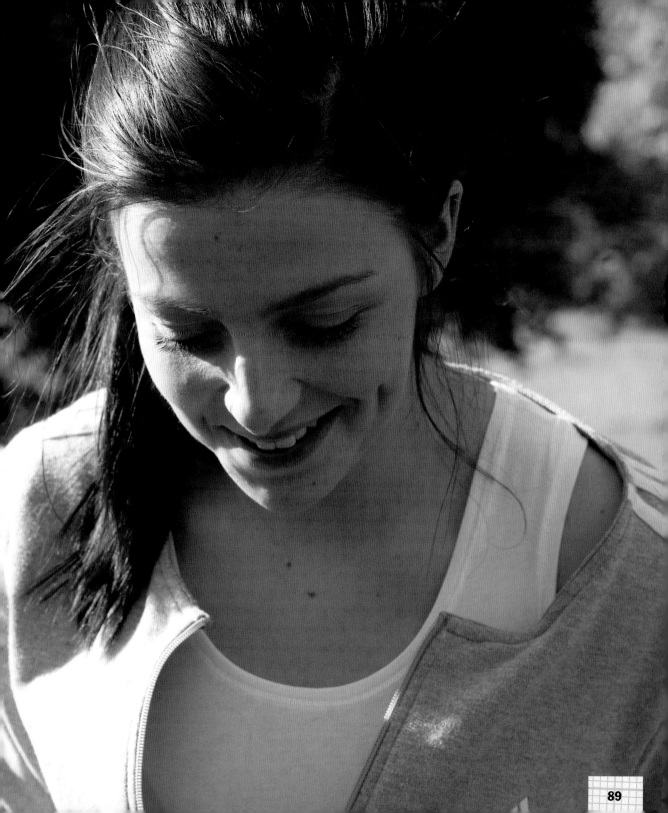

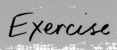
Exercise

Six kinds of exercise to try	
Yoga	Good for flexibility as well as for giving your mind a break. There are as many different types of yoga as there are personality types, from calm Hatha yoga to energetic Ashtanga yoga, so there will be one that suits you.
Wall-climbing	Great for developing strength in a wide variety of muscles – and trust in your climbing partner.
Dancing	Brilliant exercise, whether you're doing aerobics classes, practising steps on a dance mat, learning to swing dance or just jumping around to your favourite songs.
Badminton	Fun to play and much more energetic than it looks.
Pilates	Brilliant for strengthening tummy muscles and very good for your posture. Find a class in your area, or borrow a pilates DVD from your local library.
Kick-boxing	Demands strength, balance and coordination. It's not aggressive when you're learning it, but it could come in handy for self-defence.

63 find ways to stay motivated

Joining a team is a good way to get to know other people. School teams often get to go on great trips, too. Exercising with a friend means that even if you don't feel like doing whatever you had planned, you won't want to let your exercise buddy down. Doing exercise for charity gives you a goal to train towards. Find out if there's a sponsored walk, run, or swim that you could sign up for – then you'll be helping a good cause, too.

64 wear a sports bra

When you exercise, you should wear a sports bra to support your breasts properly and minimize the amount that they move. If your breasts are constantly bouncing around, the ligaments that hold them in place will become stretched and, over the years, that will make them sag.

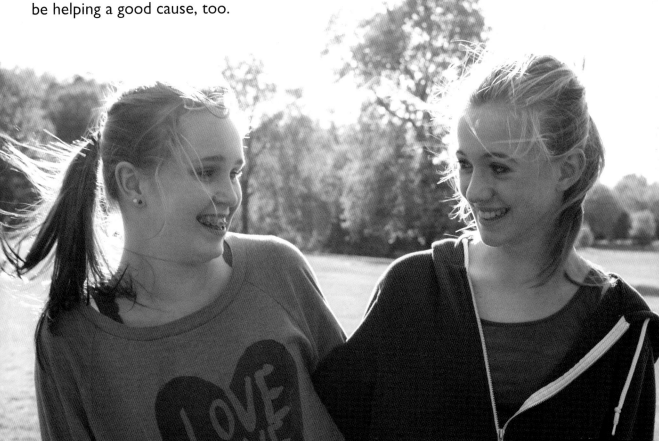

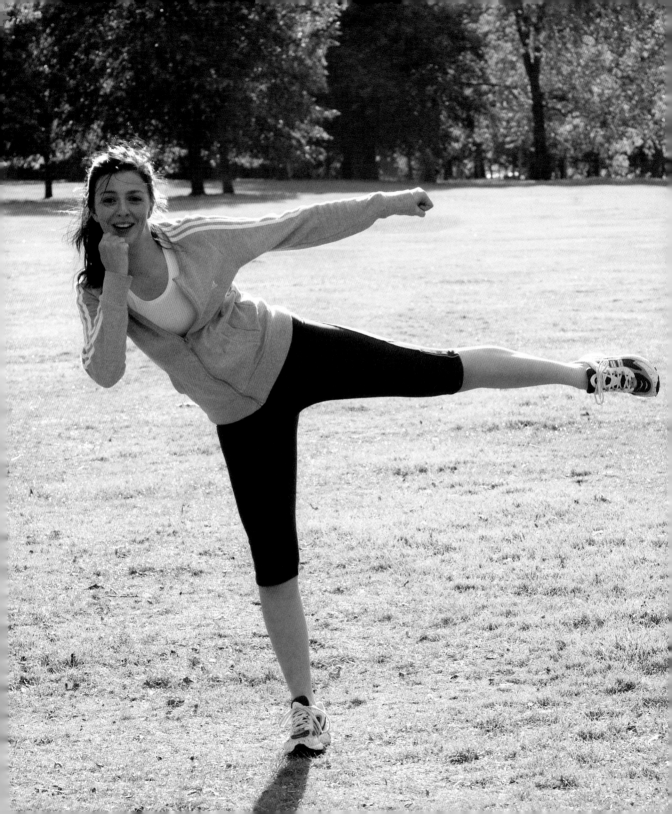

65 take an all-round approach to fitness

There are five aspects to fitness. Ideally, you should work on all of them, rather than getting obsessed with one of them, as they all complement each other.

Flexibility

What it is: being able to stretch and bend freely in all directions.

Try: gymnastics, yoga, stretching.

Strength

What it is: training your muscles to work properly.

Try: working with weights.

Balance and coordination

What it is: teaching your body to move with grace and awareness.

Try: yoga, pilates, martial arts.

Cardiovascular fitness

What it is: getting your heart and lungs working.

Try: swimming, running or cycling.

Endurance

What it is: being able to keep going!

Try: slow, lengthy cardio exercise.

So, what is "cardio"?

The heart is the biggest muscle in the body and it needs exercise like all your other muscles. Cardio (short for "cardiovascular") or aerobic exercise is anything that raises your heart rate and gets you a bit out of breath.

As your body moves faster, your blood has to pump faster around your body in order to keep your muscles supplied with oxygen. The more cardio exercise you do, the better your heart and lungs work and the quicker your pulse rate returns to normal afterwards.

If you want to get fitter, this is the kind of exercise to do — so get your trainers or your swimming costume on and get moving.

66 learn five exercises for keeping muscles strong

These will work the main muscle groups in your legs, arms, chest, trunk and back.

Clock lunges (for legs and bum)

1. Imagine you're standing at the centre of a clock. Take a big step forward – to twelve o'clock – with your right foot, and then lower your left knee towards the ground so you're in a lunge. Return to your start position and repeat with the left leg.

2. Now step your right foot to the right – three o'clock. Sink down into a side lunge, return to the centre and repeat to the other side – nine o'clock.

3. Finally lunge your right foot backwards – to six o'clock – in a reverse lunge. Return to the centre and repeat on the left.

Row (for upper back and posture)

You can do this standing or sitting, with a stretchy band looped around a post, a tree or a friend.

1. Get a moderate tension on the band with your arms outstretched.

2. Then pull your elbows back until they are level with your waist. Squeeze the muscles in the middle of your back as you do this, and imagine you're holding a tennis ball under each armpit. Alternatively, you can do this with weights in each hand.

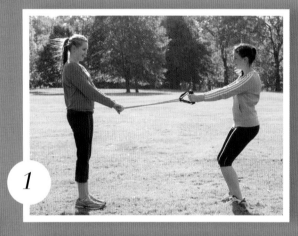

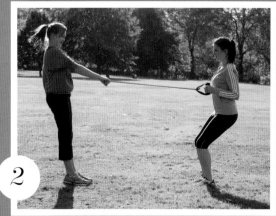

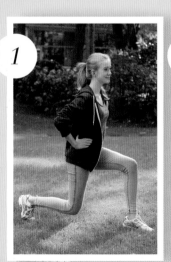

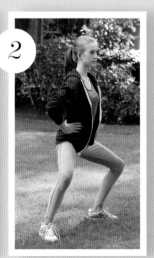

Plank – see page 98 for how to do this brilliant tummy-firming exercise.

Press-ups (for chest and tricep strength and toning)

1. Start with your knees on the floor, your ankles crossed, your hands beneath your shoulders and your arms extended. Keep your body in a straight line from your knees up to your ears.

2. Tighten your tummy muscles, squeeze your bottom muscles and lower your chest towards the ground – as close as you can go without touching dow – then push back up to the starting position. When you can do twenty easily, start in the full press-up position, on your toes rather than your knees.

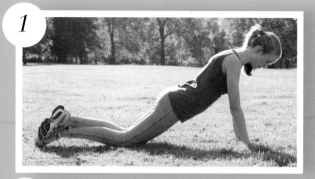

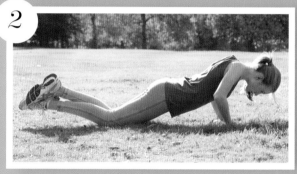

Ankle touches (for waist, tummy and neck)

1. Lie on your back with your knees bent, your feet flat on the floor, your fingers at your temples and your elbows out to the sides. Lift your head and shoulders off the ground.

2. Reach your right hand out to touch your right ankle (make sure your waist is doing the work).

3. Bring your hand back to your temple, and, still holding the sit-up position, reach your left hand to your left ankle.

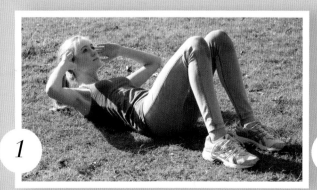

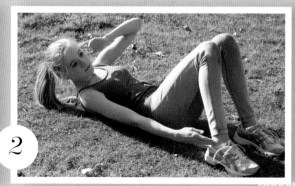

67 create a personalized exercise routine

Create your own workout by choosing exercises from the list below and mixing them up with the ones on pages 94 and 95.

If you do half of the exercises the first time, do the other half the next time. Don't just stick with the exercises you like best.

You could do each exercise ten times, or do all of them once, and then repeat the routine – it's up to you.

Cardio exercises

These exercises will get your heart pumping.

Shuttle runs

Choose two points and sprint between them, pausing for as short a time as possible each time you change direction.

Repeater step-ups

1. Stand on a step with your weight on your left foot.

2. Swing your right knee up in front of you, then reach it behind you to touch the ground. Repeat ten times then swap to the other leg.

Skipping

Do it on the spot, whirling the rope fast. It's tougher than you think!

Burpees

1. Stand tall. Jump up into the air and when you land, drop your hands to the floor with your hands by your feet.

2. Jump your feet backwards, together, into a plank position, then back up to your hands.

3. Then jump up and continue.

Boxing kicks

1. Stand with your feet hip-width apart.

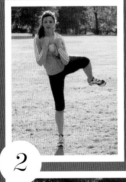

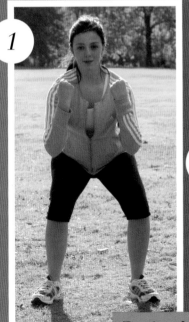

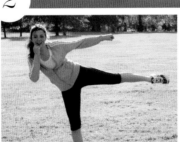

Boxing kicks

2. Drop your bum backwards in a squat, as if you were going to sit on a chair, then squeeze your bottom to move upwards again. Bring your right foot up with your right hip turned out, and extend the leg into a karate kick to the side. Repeat with the left leg.

Strength exercises

These exercises will tone your muscles.

Kettle squats

1. Stand with your feet hip-width apart, holding a weight in front of your legs in both hands. It doesn't have to be a dumbbell; a bag of rice or a bottle of water will do.

2. Sit backwards into a squat and, as you do, lift your hands and the weight up in front of you to chest height, keeping your arms straight. Once you're in the squat, push back up again and lower the weight to your thighs. Try to do the squats quite fast. Think about moving your bum backwards; it's important not to let your knees move forward over your toes.

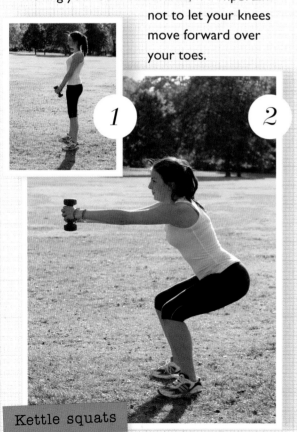

Kettle squats

Boxing

Again, this can be done with weights or a band. If you're using a band, put it behind your back, then hold it in each hand, moderately taut. Punch each hand out in front of you, aiming upwards so that when your arms are fully extended, they are at chin height.

One-leg arabesque

1. Stand on your left leg holding a weight out in front of you in both hands.

2. Bend forwards, lifting your right leg up behind you.

3. Touch the weight to the floor. Then repeat the exercise on the other leg. This is good for your bum, thighs, core strength and balance.

Knee to elbow

In full press-up position, i.e. with straight arms and legs, bend your right knee and lift it forwards towards your right elbow, without letting your bottom rise. Do as many as you can on one side, then repeat on the other. It's good for your tummy, back and shoulders.

One-leg arabesque

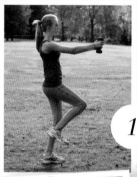

1

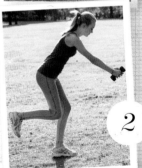

2

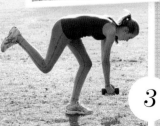

3

68 tone up your tummy

Having strong tummy muscles helps support the whole "core" of your body, this improves your posture and keeps your back strong. Strengthening your stomach muscles isn't all about crunches or sit-ups. These are the two most effective tummy-toning exercises in existence:

Plank

Lie on your front. Lift your body up so that you are resting on your forearms, with your elbows right under your shoulders. Now lift up your tummy and bottom so that there's a straight line from your shoulders to your heels. Start by holding the position for fifteen seconds and build up from there. Don't let your tummy sag – keep pulling it up and in.

Bicycle

1. Lie on your back with your knees in the air and your legs in "tabletop" position. Keep a small curve in your spine (don't push it into the ground, you want to be able to put a couple of fingers beneath your back without squishing them). Pull your tummy muscles in.

2. Put your fingertips to your temples, keeping your elbows out to the side. Lift your head and shoulders off the ground, as though you're doing a sit-up.

3. Now extend one leg out slowly and bring it back, then extend the other one, and return to the starting position. You'll feel your tummy muscles working as you do this.

4. If this feels easy, try moving both legs at the same time, like slow bicycling. Extend your right leg out slowly, bringing your left knee towards your chest at the same. While you're doing this, turn your body so your right elbow touches your left knee. Then repeat on the other side.

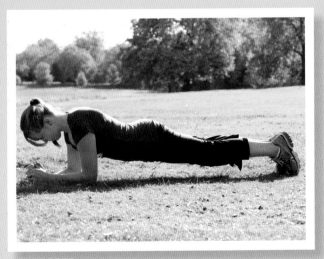

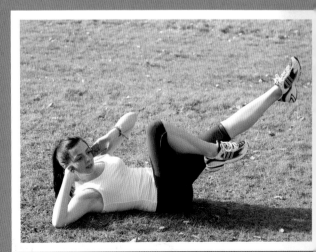

69 build up your bones

Walking, running and dancing are great for building up your bones. When you walk or run, there's a small impact each time your bodyweight hits the ground. It might not seem like much but it's enough to stimulate the osteoblasts, the cells in your bones that create new bone, into action. That's important because, in your teens, your bones are growing and becoming more dense. This bone mass will have to see you through the rest of your life, so the more you can create while you're young, the better.

tip Be consistent in your exercise routine. Yo-yo exercising – doing huge amounts of exercise and then slumping for weeks like a couch potato – is bad for the body, just like yo-yo dieting, because it's a shock to the system.

WHAT THE EXPERT SAYS

Anna Barnsley is a brilliant physiotherapist who sorts out all kinds of muscular problems. She put together the stretches and postural advice in this book. Here are her top tips:

☑ Sit and stand up properly.

This works the muscles which support and protect your joints. When you sit and stand with good posture, everything becomes easier for your body. You'll even breathe more deeply and digest your food more efficiently.

☑ Stretching is good for you.

There's endless debate about stretching – about whether it does muscles any good, and what types of stretches are best – but don't believe anyone who says stretching is pointless. Just make sure you stretch gently – your body will tell you if you're overdoing it.

☑ Do movement-based stretches just before exercise.
As a rule, the stretches I've described in these pages are great for in-between and after exercise but shouldn't be done directly before exercise. Before sport, movement-based stretching is thought to be more effective.

Exercise

70 improve your posture

Here are three good reasons why you should:

1. To stay pain free now and in the future

Standing and sitting with bad posture can lead to back and neck pain in later life. The human skeleton is designed to walk and run, so move around when you can.

2. Standing and sitting well makes life a bit less of an effort

Sitting in a way that's comfortable for your body uses up less energy, so you'll have more energy to focus on things that really matter.

3. Good posture is really important for your self-confidence

If you stand tall and look at ease in your body, other people will automatically think that you're a relaxed, confident person, even if you don't feel it yourself. In the same way that forcing a smile can actually make you feel happier, assuming a confident way of standing or walking can actually affect the way you feel about yourself, and make you feel more confident, too.

tip Don't cross your legs. You hardly notice, but crossing your legs twists your pelvis slightly and over time it can create muscle tension and make you a little wonky.

71 stand up straight

Yes, yes, we all know how to stand up straight ... but this is how to tweak yourself into line so a physiotherapist would approve.

1. Stand with your weight evenly distributed on both feet. Your feet should be about shoulder-width apart, so your feet are under your hips, and turned out very slightly (about fifteen degrees).

2. Two-thirds of your weight should be on your heels.

3. Keep your knees soft – don't brace them backwards or "lock" them.

4. Gently squeeze in your bottom muscles.

5. Lengthen through the upper back as if someone is pulling you up with a piece of string through the top of the head (your collarbone will lift slightly).

6. Drop your shoulders back and down. Don't pull your shoulders back, military style – it's not natural, it creates tension in your back and shoulders and it's not "functional" – you can't hold that position and use your arms in a normal way.

7. Finally, gently tuck your chin in slightly. If someone is looking at you from the side, there should be a straight line from your shoulders to your knees, running through your hips and slightly behind your knees.

72 sit in the right position

It's not just about sitting up straight…

1. Tuck your feet slightly underneath you so that your knees are lower than your hips and make sure your weight is equally distributed on both seat bones.

2. Lengthen through the upper back.

3. Drop your shoulders.

4. Tuck your chin in very slightly (try to avoid sticking your chin forward like a tortoise poking its head out of its shell).

5. If you are looking at a computer screen, the top of the screen should be directly level with your eyes as you look straight ahead in your good sitting position.

Did you know?
When you sit down, about eight times your bodyweight pushes down through your pelvis, compressing it. Loosen things up by dancing around your bedroom, classroom or kitchen every so often. It's a good way to stimulate your brain, too.

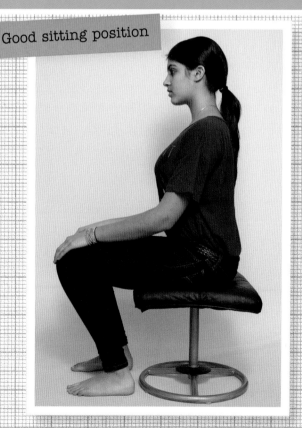

Good sitting position

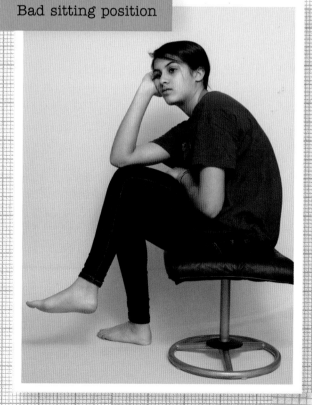

Bad sitting position

73 stretch your muscles

In your teens, your bones grow really quickly, and your muscles can't always keep up. Too much sitting down doesn't help – it encourages your muscles to stay short and tight. Stretching your muscles makes them longer and loosens them up.

Stretching muscles is not like stretching a jumper that has shrunk in the wash and only needs a few short tugs to get it back into shape. In order to stimulate your muscles to lengthen, you need them to send lots of repeated, regular messages to the brain that they're too short. The key is to stretch often, not just before or after sport.

The most important stretches

Hold each stretch for twenty seconds and repeat them as often as you can. If any of your muscles are really short, the ideal way to work them is to stretch them six times a day. To start with, pick a couple of stretches to work on. When they get easier, add others.

Calves

Your calf muscles get very tight, especially if you're starting to wear shoes with high heels.

1. Facing a wall, lean onto it with both hands.

2. Extend one leg out behind you, keeping the heel on the floor. Feel the stretch in the calf.

3. Bend your front knee and keep a straight slope from your shoulders to your heel.

4. Repeat with the other leg.

Chest

Great for preventing rounded shoulders.

1. Stand facing a wall.

2. Place your right hand on the wall, level with your shoulder. Keeping your arm straight, roll your right shoulder back.

3. Slowly turn to the left, walking your feet around as you go. Feel the stretch in the muscles on the right of your chest.

4. Turn around to repeat on your left side.

Neck

This is a good one to do every half an hour while you're studying to release tension.

1. In a good sitting posture, place your right hand behind your back.

2. Take your left hand over the top of your head, wrapping your fingers over to hold the head just behind the right ear.

3. Gently pull the head to the left and slightly forwards, as if you're looking under your left armpit. Feel the stretch down your neck and into the right shoulder.

4. Repeat on the opposite side.

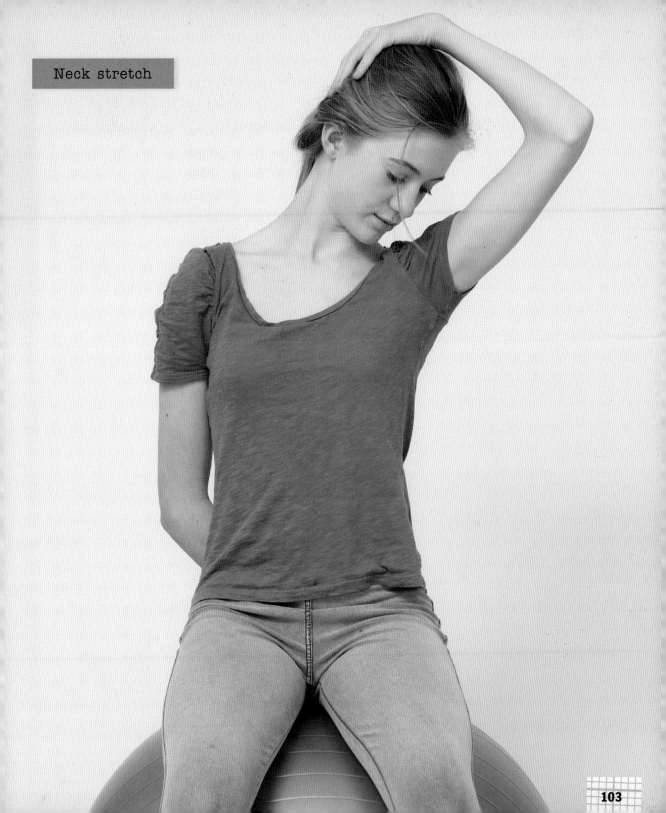

Neck stretch

Mid-back, chest and arm stretch

This really stretches your back and chest and strengthens your tummy and bottom at the same time.

1. Lie in a bridge position over a gym ball (sometimes called a Swiss Ball) with your back on the ball. Make sure your bottom is lifted and gently squeezed in.

2. Take your arms out to your side, palms up. Feel the stretch in your chest, arms and upper back.

3. Repeat with the arms above the head, first with the palms up and then with the thumbs pointing down.

Hamstring stretch

Hamstrings run down the backs of your legs and tend to be the worst culprits in terms of shortening. If you can't touch your toes, your hamstrings are too short.

1. Lie on your back, with one leg straight out on the floor and the other leg bent.

2. Using both hands, pull the bent leg towards you.

3. Bring your toes towards you, slowly straightening the leg at the knee until you feel a stretch behind the thigh.

4. Repeat with the other leg.

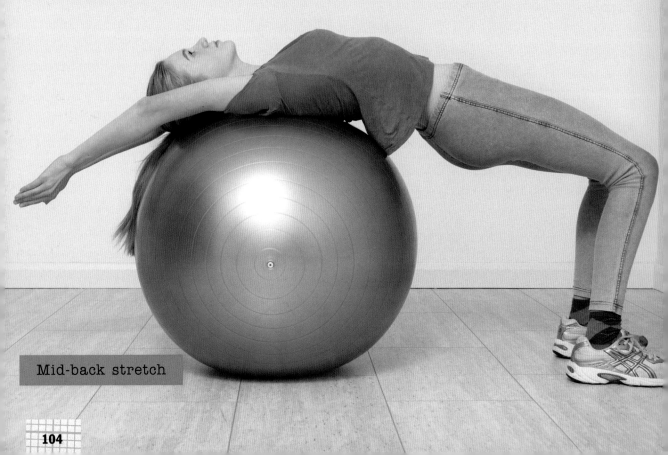

Mid-back stretch

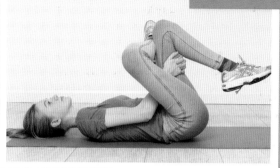

Glute stretch

Quadricep stretch

Your quadriceps are the big muscles at the front of the thighs. They get used all the time and really benefit from regular stretching.

1. Stand tall, then (using a wall, chair or table if you need help balancing), bend one knee and lift your heel up behind you towards your bottom and take hold of your ankle. Keep your knees together and your hips pushed forwards while you do this. Feel the stretch in the front of the thigh.

2. Repeat with the other leg.

Glute stretch

The big gluteal muscles in your bottom get used all the time, especially in sport.

1. Lie on your back with your knees bent and your feet flat on the floor.

2. Put your right ankle on your left thigh, near the knee, and drop your right knee out to the side.

3. Reach behind your left thigh and pull this – and your right ankle, with it – towards your face, and feel the stretch in your right buttock.

4. Swap sides and stretch the left glute.

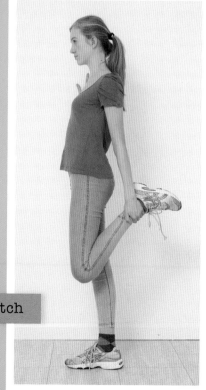

Quadricep stretch

Beth on growing pains

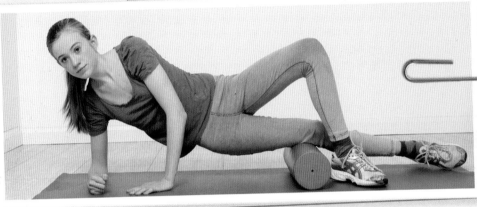

Q So, do you stretch?

A I do now! Last year my knees were really painful and I couldn't work out what was causing it, so I went to see a physiotherapist. She told me my knees were hurting because I had a condition called Osgood-Schlatter disease, where you have a growth spurt and the bones in your legs grow faster than the muscles do. That means the muscles are stretched really tightly, especially around the joints like the knees, so when I bent my knees, it really hurt. She said a lot of people probably have this but don't realize why their knees are hurting.

Q So what did you have to do?

A I had to learn stretches to lengthen the muscles down the front of the thigh, the back of the thigh and the back of the calves, rolling them over a hard foam roller. The stretches really hurt – but in a way that I know is doing me good – and if I do them regularly, twice a day, my knees are much more comfortable than if I don't.

Wellbeing

Your mood, your self-esteem
and what you eat are all connected.
Choosing the right foods will make you feel
calmer and happier, and feeling great will
boost your confidence so you can get on with
the things that really matter in your life.

WHAT THE EXPERT SAYS

Nina Grunfeld always spent a lot of time helping people find their purpose in life. Now it is her career. Her latest book, *How to Get What You Want*, is written especially for young adults. Here are her top tips:

☑ **Try new things.** Everything you do will build your confidence. So keep doing things, meeting people, trying new adventures.

☑ **Accept who you are.** Treat yourself as you would a best friend. Don't compare yourself to others – you're unique!

☑ **Know yourself.** Every day, ask yourself what the best thing that happened to you that day was. Notice what you like and dislike, what makes you happy and what makes you sad. This will help you make decisions that are right for you.

☑ **Do something you want to do every day.** Notice how much you're achieving and congratulate yourself.

☑ **Be nice to yourself.** You talk to yourself more than anyone else does. Think and say positive things to yourself.

74 think positive

The way you think affects the way you feel – and it affects the people around you, too. Negative thoughts – that everything is going wrong, that you are no good – drag you down. Positive thoughts – that things are great, that you're doing just fine – make you feel happy and well. You may not realize it, but the way you think is up to you.

The habit of happiness

Thinking positively is something you can learn to do. OK, it's not easy, but if you catch yourself feeling negative, tell yourself to stop and try looking at things another way. Positive thinking is a habit and, like other habits, it needs a bit of work to make it stick.

Try visualization: think ahead about an event that's coming up, as if you're watching a film of it in your mind. Imagine everything going really well. You'll feel much more confident and better prepared if you run through the event in your mind.

75 be grateful

It's easy to find things to complain about in life. What's harder, but much more rewarding in the long-term, is to think about the best things in your life and feel grateful for them. Try doing this every evening.

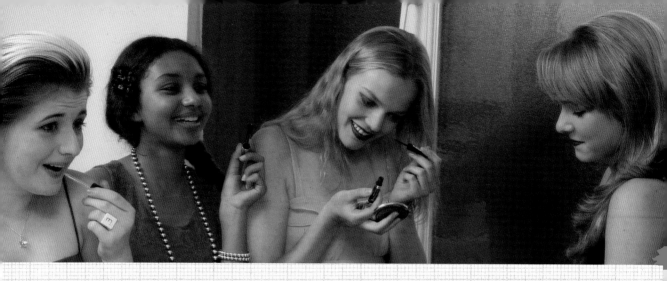

76 be your own best friend

To have good self-esteem, you have to like yourself. You need to be your own best friend before you let anyone else join in. If you feel that you don't like yourself that much, try giving yourself regular compliments, particularly when you do something well.

77 be proud of who you are

However much we like to belong to a group (and we do, it's the way we're made), we're all different. You need to learn to value the things that set you apart from everyone else. Once you really value yourself and your unique qualities, your path in life becomes that little bit easier.

78 remember it's beauty on the inside that counts

Yes, it's fun playing around with clothes, make-up and hairstyles, and trying to look our best. But don't forget that it's who you are on the inside that really matters.

79 don't follow the herd

It may seem easier, or safer, to do what everyone else is doing – to dress, think, or behave in the same way. But you don't have to. The better you know yourself, the easier it will be to strike out on your own. Just because everyone else is acting a certain way doesn't meant that it's right – or that it's right for you.

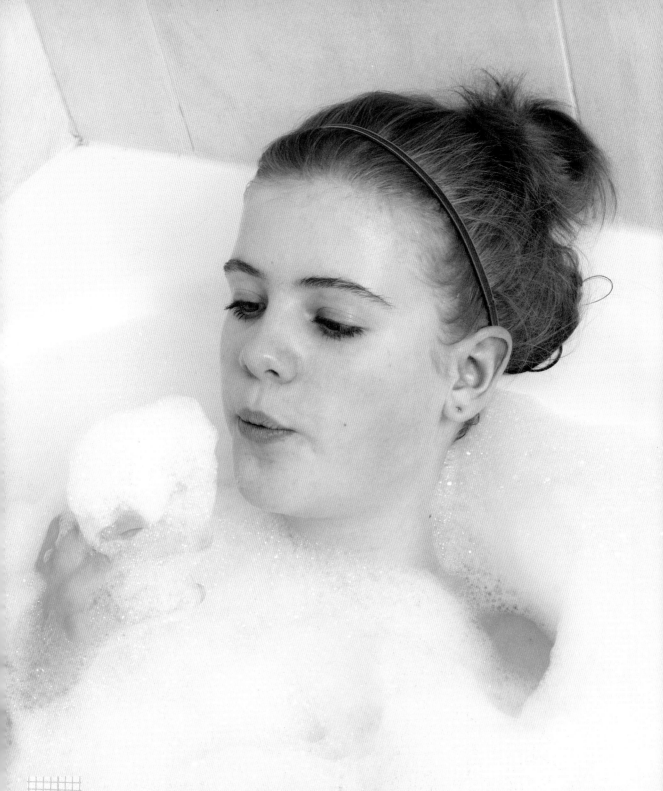

80 find ways to relax

Relaxing and taking it easy is really good for you. It helps to put things in perspective when life, family, friends or schoolwork are getting too much. Different things work for different people. You could always sit down in front of the TV, but here are some other ideas to try.

Relaxation ideas

❤ Do some gentle exercise – go for a swim, or a long walk.

❤ Chill out to soothing music.

❤ Play with a pet – walk your dog, or someone else's.

❤ Dance to loud music.

❤ Get into the kitchen and get cooking.

❤ Take a long bath.

These are also great ways to cheer yourself up when you're feeling down.

81 breathe deeply

Taking slow, deep breaths is really good for your mind as well as your body. As toddlers, we all automatically breathe steadily and deeply, and our stomachs rise and fall as we do. As we grow up, we lose this habit and start breathing more shallowly – but if you take the time to relax and breathe deeply once in a while, your body and brain will really thank you for it.

An easy breathing exercise

1. Lie down with your legs bent and your feet resting on the floor.

2. Rest your hands on your stomach and breathe, slowly and deeply, into your stomach, so that your hands rise. Don't push the breath or force it, just let it happen.

3. Breathe out slowly, and notice your hands fall back to where they were.

4. As you breathe, relax, and try to just observe your breath. Imagine your breath as a long stream of silver ribbon that you're breathing in, then breathing out.

5. Do this ten times. If you have time, try doing three rounds of ten breaths.

tip It doesn't particularly matter whether you breathe through your nose or mouth. Try breathing in through your nose and out through your mouth, to give you something to focus on.

82 go to bed super-early once a week

Sleep is really important. While you're asleep, your body releases a hormone that's essential for all the growing that your body is doing. It's better to go to bed early rather than sleeping late in the morning – sleep experts say every hour's sleep before midnight is worth two hours afterwards. Give it a try.

83 break it down

Try this when you've got to do something that seems too huge to manage and you feel overwhelmed.

There's a popular joke in self-help circles which goes:

**Q "How do you eat an elephant?"
A "Bit by bit."**

The point is that if you look at a problem as a whole, whether it's clearing up a messy bedroom or revising all your subjects for exams, it can seem overwhelming. If you split the task into smaller chunks and make a plan to tackle these one by one, it's much easier to manage.

84 practise being happy

It sounds strange, but happiness is something that can be worked on.

Imagine that an outing you were looking forward to gets cancelled. Do you:

a) Shout and scream?

b) Feel down and spend the rest of the day blaming other people for anything and everything?

c) Feel disappointed, but get over it, and find something else to do instead?

It's just like thinking positively (page 108) – you can decide for yourself to have that third response. Lots of things that you can't control may well affect how you feel, but if you make a conscious effort to change your thoughts and behaviour, you can change the way you feel, too.

85 smile

You probably know the saying, "smile and the world smiles with you". When you smile, even if you're forcing it, you automatically feel happier, because the action releases endorphins, the body's feel-good chemicals. If you approach people with a smile, you'll feel better, and it might put a smile on their faces, too.

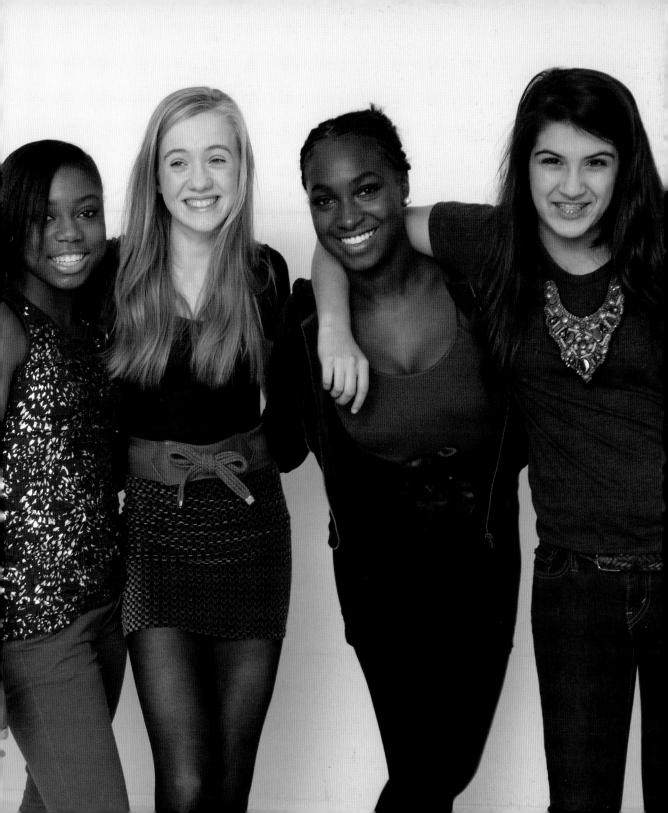

86 keep talking to your parents

You're growing up and becoming independent. It's unavoidable that you'll have differences of opinion with your parents. However much you feel that they don't understand you, remember that they love you greatly and will always be prepared to talk to you – if you give them the chance. It's more than likely that once, way back in the mists of time, they went through something similar to what you're going through.

87 do as you would be done by

It's an old-fashioned idea, but one which everyone would do well to bear in mind. It means that you should behave towards other people as you would like them to behave towards you. The world would be a much better place if everyone followed this advice.

88 do what you love

Finding your sense of self and your own way in life is tricky. Often, friends and family will try to influence you one way or another – to study the same subject as them, or to like the same sports or hobbies that they like. Doing what you want rather than what others want you to do may not be easy, but it will make you happier in the long term.

89 beat your inner critic

We've all got one, that little voice somewhere at the back of our minds. It pops up, usually when we're feeling tired, ill or down, telling us that in one way or another we're not good enough. If you find yourself thinking negative thoughts, tell your inner critic to take a back seat and give yourself a positive compliment instead. Focusing on the good things in your day can help keep your inner critic quiet and put you in a better mood.

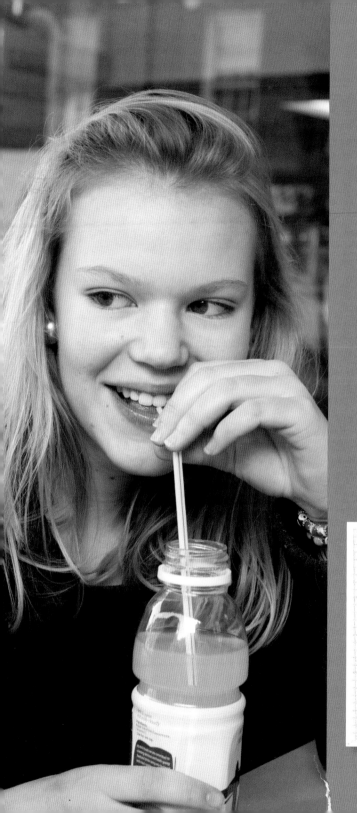

90 eat yourself happy

Not by using food to comfort yourself, but by knowing which foods have a positive effect on your mood and feeling of wellbeing (and no, sugar isn't one of them). Cakes might seem comforting but that's only in the short-term, until the sugar high wears off.

You probably already have a fair idea of what's good for you (meat, fish, eggs, vegetables, fruit, milk, cheese, yogurt, wholemeal bread) and what isn't (sugar, biscuits, doughnuts, crisps, takeaways, chips, fizzy drinks). Aim to base your meals on healthy foods and keep the other stuff for occasional indulgence.

Good-mood foods

♥ Oily fish, nuts, seeds (for all those healthy omega oils).

♥ Wholegrains and green vegetables (for B-vitamins and steady energy release).

♥ Eggs, meat, fish, cheese, pulses (for the protein they contain, which provides tryptophan, an amino-acid that is known as a mood balancer).

WHAT THE EXPERT SAYS

What leading nutritionist Ian Marber doesn't know about food and vitamins and what they can do for you is hardly worth knowing. Here are his top tips:

☑ **Make sure you eat enough.**
Weight management isn't about starving yourself. If you don't eat enough, your body thinks that you're in a famine. The moment you eat a little more, and you will because you'll be too hungry not to, your body stores the extra away ready for the next famine.

☑ **Don't count calories.** Thinking about food in terms of calories is misleading. Foods that help you have great skin, hair, energy and a good mood may not be the lowest in calories.

☑ **Eat little and often.** Eating small amounts throughout the day keeps your metabolism ticking over nicely, so eat breakfast, a small snack, lunch, another snack in the afternoon and then dinner.

☑ **Eat complex carbohydrates with protein.** Foods are broken down in the digestive system at different speeds and, in order to supply the body with consistent energy, you need to combine the food groups.

91 cut out sugar

If you want to improve your health by doing just one thing, give up refined sugar and foods that contain it.

Why sugar is bad for you

Yes, sugar gives you energy, but all food gives you energy. Sugar just gives you an instant glucose rush which your body struggles to sort out. As well as keeping your blood sugar levels more steady, avoiding sugar can help keep your skin clear. Dermatologists have noted the links between high sugar consumption and acne, though no one has fully explained how the two are connected.

92 pass on junk food

That means avoiding processed food, takeaways and ready meals as much as possible. Of course, if someone is having a pizza party, you'll want to join in, but where you have a choice over what you eat, go for cooked-from-scratch options made with wholesome, fresh ingredients.

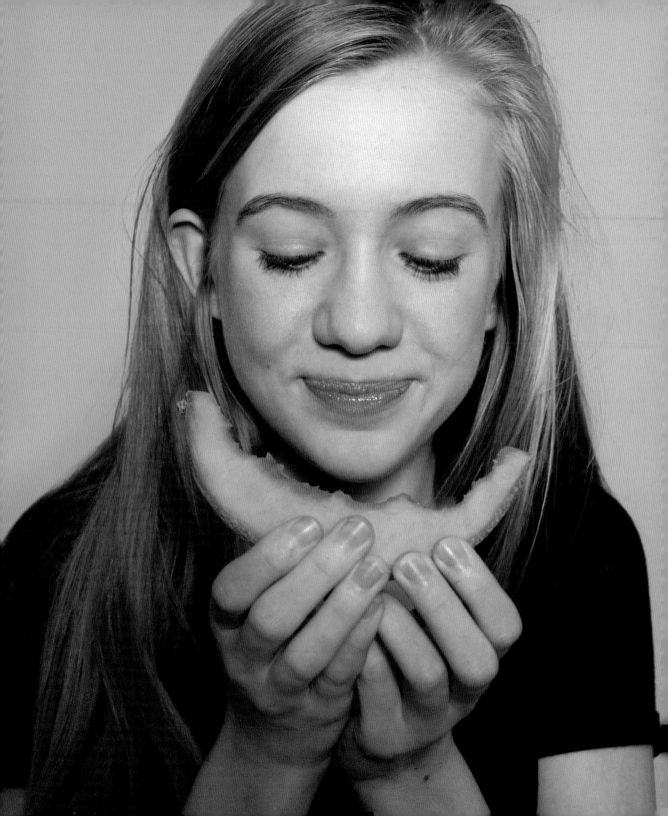

93 get enough essential fats

Get your head around the fact that fat is good for you — especially omega-3 essential fatty acids, which you find in oily fish, seeds and some nuts.

These fatty acids are called "essential" because they're crucial in keeping your body healthy but your body can't make them for itself. They keep your brain and heart healthy, your mood level, and your skin, hair and nails looking good.

94 keep up the calcium

Your body needs plenty of calcium in order to make strong bones. Milk, cheese and yogurt are all full of calcium. If you aren't eating much in the way of dairy products, other good

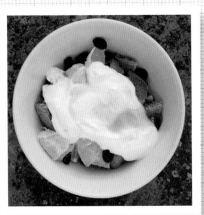

sources of calcium include seeds, green vegetables like cabbage and broccoli, sardines and tofu.

95 aim for a rainbow plate

The best way to get the nutrients you need is to choose foods from every colour of the rainbow — especially brightly coloured fruit and vegetables. We're talking naturally red strawberries, purple aubergines and yellow peppers here, not artificially coloured cereals or sweets. Make sure the carbohydrates you eat are brown (wholegrain) rather than white, too.

Why fruit, vegetables and wholegrains are good for you

Fruits and vegetables are full of antioxidants, which are thought to protect your body's cells. Fruit and veg are a good source of fibre, too, which helps keep your digestive system healthy.

Wholemeal bread and brown rice and pasta are better choices than their white or "refined" equivalents. Wholegrain options contain more vitamins and fibre than their refined cousins, so they keep you full for longer and are more nutritious.

tip Don't get hung up on having skimmed milk rather than whole milk. High-fat foods are those which are 20% fat, and high-fat liquid foods are 10% fat. Full-fat milk is only 4% fat.

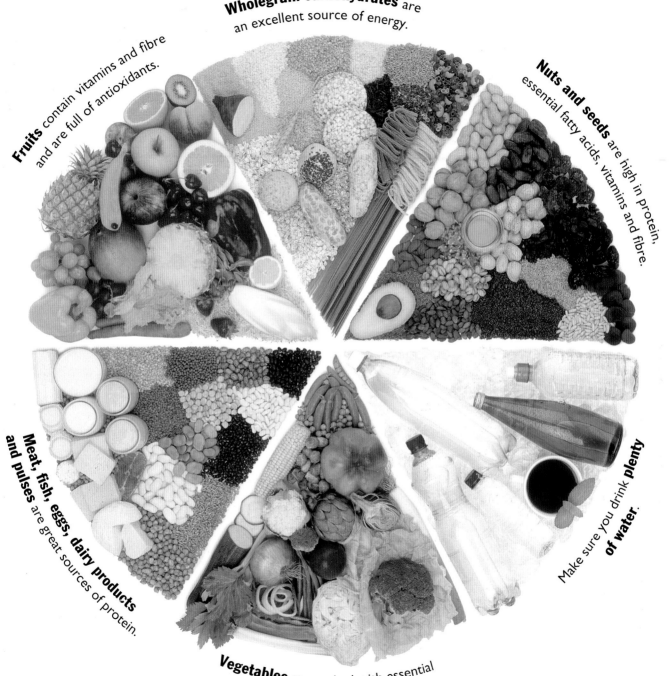

Wholegrain carbohydrates are an excellent source of energy.

Fruits contain vitamins and fibre and are full of antioxidants.

Nuts and seeds are high in protein, essential fatty acids, vitamins and fibre.

Meat, fish, eggs, dairy products and pulses are great sources of protein.

Make sure you drink **plenty of water**.

Vegetables are packed with essential vitamins and fibre.

Wellbeing

96 get enough vitamins

You can find most of the vitamins and minerals you need in food if you know where to look. You'd think you could just take a vitamin pill and have done with it, but the body doesn't absorb vitamins from pills as well as it does from food. You're better off eating well rather than eating rubbish and hoping that vitamin pills will make up for it. If anything needs supplementing it is omega-3 essential fatty acids, which you find in fish oil supplements.

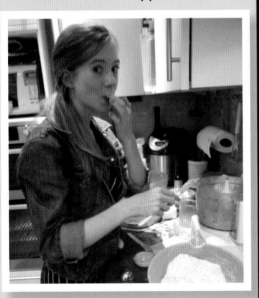

Vitamin/mineral	Why do you need it?
Iron	Iron is needed to make red blood cells and carry oxygen around your body. If you're short of iron, you become anaemic. You look pale, feel tired and can't concentrate properly. Girls need more iron than boys because menstruation reduces your iron levels.
Calcium	To build strong bones.
Vitamin D	To keep your bones strong and your immune system working well.
Essential fatty acids	To keep your brain, skin and heart in best shape.
Zinc	To boost immunity, heal wounds and digest food properly.

Where can you get it naturally?	How much should you have?	Is it worth taking a supplement?
The best source is red meat. You also find iron in dried fruit, fortified breakfast cereals, bread and green leafy vegetables, though the body doesn't absorb iron so well from these. Having some vitamin C at the same time helps improve absorption.	Teenage girls need around 15 mg of iron a day.	It is if you're vegetarian or if you don't eat much of the foods that contain iron. Around one in four teenage girls is anaemic.
Milk, cheese, yogurt and green leafy vegetables.	Teenagers need around 800 – 1000 mg of calcium a day. Three portions of dairy food – e.g. a yogurt, a glass of milk (or milk on cereal) and a chunk of cheese – should do the trick.	You shouldn't need to – it's not difficult to eat enough calcium.
The body makes its own vitamin D when the summer sun shines on your skin.	Exposing your hands, face and arms to sunlight for a few minutes several times a week is enough – but make sure you remember your sunscreen.	May be worth taking in the winter. Vitamin D is stored in the body so you build up supplies during the summer, but by spring most of us have low levels.
Oily fish such as mackerel, salmon, sardines and halibut, and pumpkin and flax seeds.	Oily fish once or twice a week, or as many pumpkin seeds as you like.	Yes, most of us are short of these.
Cheese, meat, shellfish, seeds and beans.	You don't need much – a handful of sunflower seeds each day is plenty.	If you have white flecks in your nails, yes (because that's a sign you're short of zinc).

97 drink plenty of water

You don't have to glug it until you slosh, but your body needs decent amounts of water to function, to exercise and to keep your brain working at its best. Water is good for you – much better than fizzy drinks and fruit juices, not to mention cheaper.

Drinks to limit

♦ **Fizzy drinks** are loaded with sugar. Diet fizzy drinks make your body think it's getting something sweet. When it doesn't, it makes you crave sweet things to make up for what it thought it was getting. Both types can deplete your body of calcium, which means you can't build strong bones.

♦ **Fruit juices** contain high levels of sugar. And a few vitamins, yes, but mostly sugar.

♦ **Caffeinated drinks** give you a buzz, but lead to an energy drop afterwards as your body re-balances itself.

98 learn to cook

Get to grips with a few basic recipes – whether it's omelettes, or a simple chilli con carne – so you can cook wholesome food and show off your skills to your friends.

99 always eat breakfast

By the morning, your system is running on empty. Your body needs refuelling and your brain needs energy in order to concentrate on school work. If you can't face eating scrambled eggs on toast (an ideal breakfast), you could always whizz up some yogurt, porridge oats, frozen berries and some seeds or nuts into a smoothie. Cereals like porridge and plain Weetabix and Shreddies make a sustaining breakfast, especially if you add protein in the form of chopped nuts. Toast or cereal is better than nothing, but most breakfast cereals are loaded with sugar and will leave you feeling hungry by mid-morning.

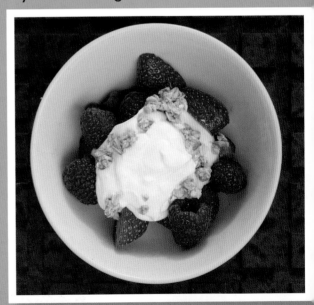

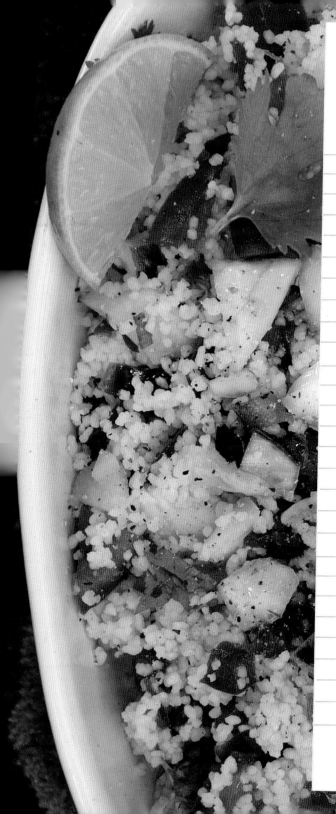

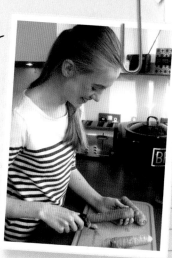

Beth on healthy eating

Q Do you find it hard to eat healthily?

A No – as long as there's healthy food on offer at mealtimes! I try to have healthy snacks like nuts or fruit instead of chocolate, cake and crisps, and not eat puddings too often.

Q Are you a fussy eater?

A I used to be, but I'm not really any more, and I try new foods whenever I get the chance. I like some things now that I never used to like – I used to hate salmon until I found a recipe for fishcakes, which are delicious.

Q Do you like cooking?

A Yes! And if I'm the one cooking the meal, I can leave out any ingredients I don't like, or try cooking things in different ways. Cooking with other people is fun, too, and I like learning other people's ways of doing things.

100 have fun!

Be your own fabulous self ... and enjoy every minute of it.

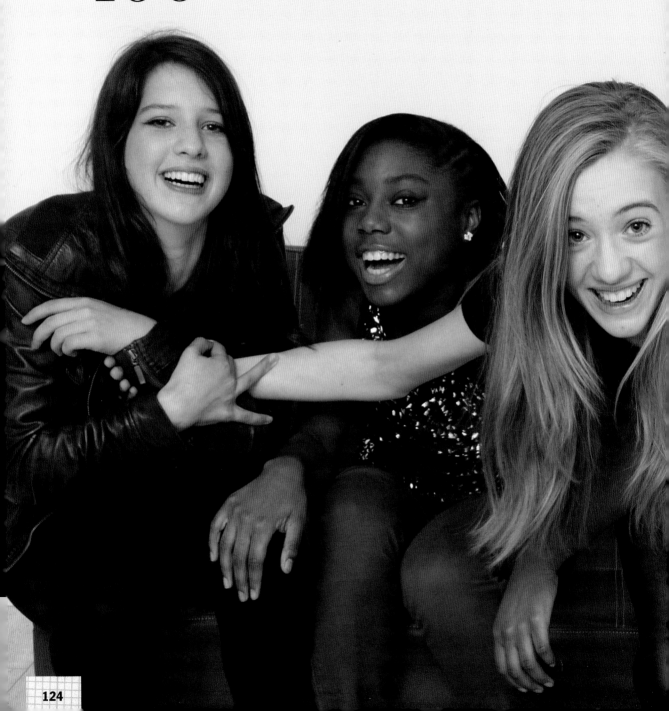

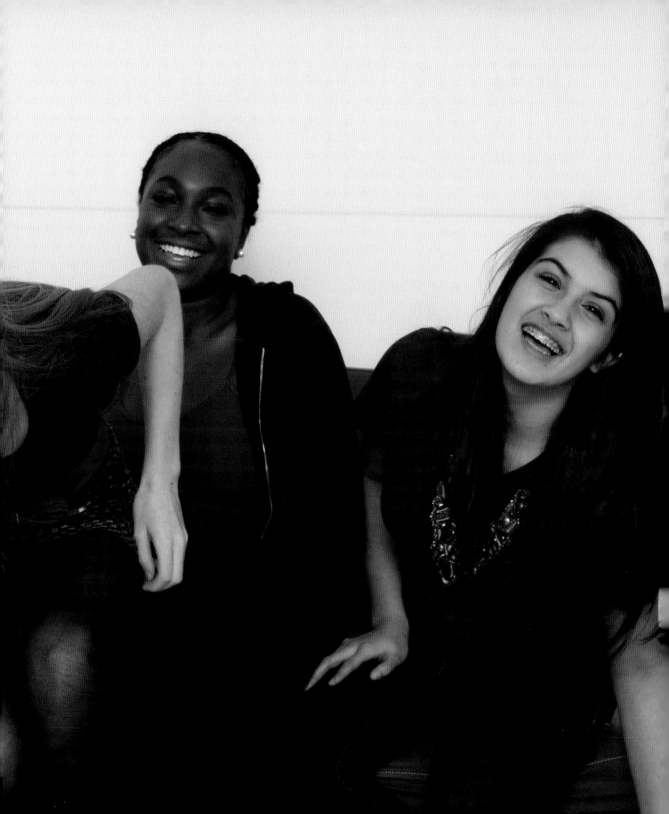

Index

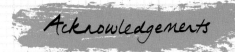
Acknowledgements

Alice and Beth would like to thank:
The wonderful team at Walker Books:
Denise Johnstone-Burt, Louise Jackson,
Charlie Moyler, Ellen Holgate and
Kate Davies;

Suki Dhanda and her assistant Laura McCluskey
for the fab photos: www.sukidhanda.com;

Louise Constad and Eleanor Andrews
for their inspired make-up:
www.beautyqueenworkshops.com;

Mathew Alexander and Sophie Bremner
for the spectacular hairstyles:
www.mathewalexander.co.uk;

Kathryn Freeland for putting the girls
through their paces in the park:
www.absolutefitness.co.uk;

Our gorgeous models Avery, Daisy, Divya, Eliza F,
Eliza P, Ella Rose, Emily E, Emily M, Evie, Georgia,
Grace, Helena, Latoya, Laura, Monique,
Suki and last but not least, Molly;

WAH Nails for the stunning nail-art photographs:
www.wah-nails.com;

Nail Rock for the nail wrap photograph:
www.nailrock.com;

We are hugely grateful to all the specialists who
have so kindly given us their time and expertise:

Dr Sam Bunting, dermatologist: 020 7467 8533;

Shavata Singh, eyebrow-shaping specialist:
www.shavata.co.uk;

Andrea Fulerton, celebrity nail technician:
www.andreafulerton.com;

Dr Uchenna Okoye, aesthetic dentist:
www.londonsmiling.com;

Lynnette Peck Bateman, style journalist and vintage
clothing specialist:
www.lovelysvintageemporium.com;

Dr Jennifer Jones, consultant dermatologist,
Royal Free Hospital;

Nina Grunfeld, founder of lifeclubs:
www.lifeclubs.co.uk;

Anna Barnsley, physiotherapist:
www.annabarnsleyphysio.co.uk;

Ian Marber, nutritionist and author:
www.ianmarber.com.

And, as always, to Matthew and Robert for their
support and good humour.

Disclaimer:

The content of this book is not intended as medical
advice and is provided for informational purposes only.
If in doubt, please consult a health care professional.

First published 2012 by Walker Books Ltd
87 Vauxhall Walk, London SE11 5HJ

10 9 8 7 6 5 4 3 2 1

Text © 2012 Alice Hart-Davis and Beth Hindhaugh

Photographs © 2009, 2012 Walker Books Ltd,
Photographs by Suki Dhanda except nail-art photographs
(pages 58-59) © Alex Sainsbury/ WAH Nails and nail wrap
photograph (page 57) © Nail Rock

Illustrations © 2012 Miminne

The right of Alice Hart-Davis and Beth Hindhaugh to
be identified as authors of this work has been asserted
by them in accordance with the Copyright, Designs and
Patents Act 1988

This book has been typeset in Gill Sans

Printed in China

British Library Cataloguing in Publication Data:
a catalogue record for this book is available
from the British Library

ISBN 978-1-4063-3754-9

www.walker.co.uk